SEDATION, ANESTHESIA,

and

the JCAHO

Second Edition

Dean F. Smith, MD

OPUS COMMUNICATIONS
A Division of *hc*Pro

Sedation, Anesthesia, and the JCAHO, Second Edition, is published by
Opus Communications, Inc., a subsidiary of HCPro Corp.

Copyright 2001 by Opus Communications, Inc., a subsidiary of HCPro Corp.

ISBN 1-57839-114-8

Opus Communications provides informational resources for the healthcare industry.
A selected listing of our newsletters and other books is found in the back of this book.

Neither HCPro Corp. nor Opus Communications, Inc., is affiliated in any way with the
Joint Commission on Accreditation of Healthcare Organizations.

Dean F. Smith, MD, Author
Karin Commeret, Managing Editor
Gillian Buckley, Associate Publisher
Suzanne Perney, Publisher
Feroza Unvala, CLYF Communications, Cover Designer and Graphic Artist
Mike Mirabello, Production
Jean St. Pierre, Creative Director

For more information, contact:

Opus Communications
PO Box 1168
Marblehead, MA 01945
Telephone: 800/650-6787 or 781/639-1872
Fax: 781/639-2982
E-mail: customer_service@hcpro.com
Website: www.hcmarketplace.com or www.hcpro.com

Contents

About the Author iv

Acknowledgments v

Preface to the Second Edition vii

Introduction ix

Chapter 1: Anesthesia and Sedation 1

Chapter 2: The JCAHO's New Sedation-
and Anesthesia-Related Standards 11

Chapter 3: Credentialing and Privileging Requirements 79

Chapter 4: The JCAHO Survey 91

Chapter 5: Performance Monitoring and Improvement . . . : 105

Appendix A: Sample Sedation Policy and Consent Forms 121

Appendix B: Anesthesia Guidelines and Standards 139

Appendix C: Sample Educational Material 163

About the Author

Dean F. Smith, MD, is board certified in anesthesiology and pediatrics. He is in private practice in pediatric anesthesiology with Valley Anesthesiology Consultants, Ltd., in Phoenix, Arizona. Dr. Smith is the past chairman of anesthesia and the current president of the medical staff at St. Joseph's Hospital and Medical Center in Phoenix.

Acknowledgments

The author gratefully acknowledges the technical assistance, skills, and patience of Karin Commeret, Kim McTighe Smith, RN, Jan Magallanez, RN, Patricia Durlam, RN, John Bull, MD, Theresa Garcia, and Ginny Blossom. Thanks also to Courtney, Matt, and Mallory Smith for their patience and support.

The author also would like to thank John Rosing, Gillian Buckley, Richard Alexander, MD, Pamela Avery, MD, Beverly Pybus, CMSC, Richard Thompson, MD, and Jack Zusman, MD, for their thoughtful reviews, suggestions, and comments. Thanks, also, to the hospitals and organizations that contributed material for this book, especially St. Joseph's Hospital and Medical Center and Catholic Healthcare West in Arizona and The Greeley Company in Marblehead, MA.

Preface to the Second Edition

For years, healthcare organizations have struggled to define *conscious sedation, anesthesia,* and *the loss of protective reflexes* in their endeavor to achieve successful JCAHO accreditation. In an attempt to provide better training, patient care, and documentation, some facilities made it their policy to apply the stricter anesthesia standards to conscious sedation, thus simplifying processes and creating greater expectations for hospital staff and practitioners. Others developed separate conscious sedation policies that applied to cases where the "loss of protective reflexes" was not anticipated. The JCAHO considered either method of survey preparation acceptable as long as the facility could provide performance improvement data to show that patients received good care. Compliance with JCAHO standards when general anesthesia was administered was not problematic for most organizations. While most organizations had a clear understanding of what was required of them to comply with the higher-level general anesthesia standards, when it came to administering "sedation" and "conscious sedation," confusion over terms, care, and expectations was commonplace.

On January 1, 2001, the JCAHO made long-awaited revisions to its anesthesia standards. In an attempt to eliminate confusion over the term *conscious sedation* and to implement stricter expectations for patient care under these circumstances, the JCAHO implemented new standards that incorporated the definitions of sedation and anesthesia outlined by the American Society of Anesthesiologists (see pp. 140-141). The JCAHO no longer uses the phrase *loss of protective reflexes.* Instead, the new standards include definitions for three levels of sedation, as well as general anesthesia. In light of the new definitions, the term *conscious sedation*, as it was previously understood, is not used as frequently in facilities. Thus, we felt it necessary to change the title of this second edition from *Conscious Sedation, Anesthesia, and the JCAHO* to *Sedation, Anesthesia, and the JCAHO.*

It is our hope that this text will be helpful to you and your organization as you work to achieve successful JCAHO accreditation.

Introduction

In November of 1999, the Institute of Medicine, one of the four National Academies, shocked the nation with its release of *To Err Is Human: Building a Safer Healthcare System*. Amid allegations that medical errors contribute to as many as 98,000 patient deaths annually (placing medical errors as the eighth leading cause of death in the United States), widespread media response—"Medical Mistakes 8th Top Killer" in *USA Today* and "The Hazards of Hospitalization" in the *Wall Street Journal*—stirred thoughtful and emotional responses from the American medical community. Lost in the debate about the validity of the data in the IOM report was the fact that errors and accidents *do* occur in the highly complex and stressful healthcare workplace. Among the results of the report was the establishment of the federal Center for Patient Safety, as well as better reporting of adverse events and increased attention to patient safety by healthcare professionals, licensing bodies, professional societies, and the FDA.

It is worth noting that among its indictments of our healthcare system, the Institute bestowed accolades upon those who were participating in anesthesia services. According to the report, "The committee recognizes that a number of groups are already working on improving patient safety, such as the National Patient Safety Foundation and the Anesthesia Patient Safety Foundation."[1] Further, "patients who died during surgery requiring general anesthesia have been the focus of many studies over the last few decades. Anesthesia is an area in which very impressive improvements in safety have been made. As more and more

---

[1] *To Err Is Human: Building a Safer Healthcare System*, p. 6. Washington DC: National Academy Press, 2000.

attention has been focused on understanding the factors that contribute to error and on the design of safer systems, preventable mishaps have declined."[2]

Healthcare practitioners in the United States currently perform more than 25 million procedures involving anesthetics each year, as well as millions more involving sedation. In any instance, complications can occur. But even with a rapid increase in the use of anesthetics, anesthesia safety has improved dramatically over the last 40 years.[3]

There are a number of reasons for the decrease in anesthetic morbidity and mortality, including the following:

- improvements in monitoring technology, such as pulse oximetry and capnometry;
- an increase in the number of physicians who practice anesthesiology;
- better training, including simulator experience, for anesthesiologists and certified registered nurse anesthetists;
- an increase in the number of highly skilled individuals who choose to enter these fields;
- safer anesthetic agents;
- more accurate systems for delivering anesthetic agents; and
- development of and adherence to effective practice standards for perioperative care.

Nonetheless, administration of anesthesia or sedation and analgesia remain high-risk procedures. For the sake of patient safety and optimal patient outcomes, providers cannot afford to let their vigilance wane. Most anesthesia or

---

[2] *Ibid., p. 32. Washington DC: National Academy Press, 2000.*
[3] *A comprehensive review found that anesthesia-related mortality rates fell by 50–80% between 1948 and 1980 (Frederick Orkin, MD, "Practice Standards: The Midas Touch or The Emperor's New Clothes?" Anesthesiology 1989; 70: 567-71). Also, among 319,000 consecutive patients who were either healthy or had a mild systemic disease (classified by the American Society of Anesthesiologists as Physical Status I and II) and who received anesthesia at the Harvard-affiliated hospitals, there were no major preventable intra-operative injuries (John H. Eichhorn, MD, "Prevention of Intraoperative Anesthesia Accidents and Related Severe Injury Through Safety Monitoring," Anesthesiology 1989; 70: 572-7).*

sedation and analgesia is administered in facilities that are accredited by the Joint Commission on Accreditation of Healthcare Organizations (JCAHO). The information in this book is designed to help you protect patients and comply with the JCAHO standards as they relate to sedation and anesthesia.

Chapter 1 discusses when the JCAHO's sedation and anesthesia standards apply and gives basic compliance recommendations.

Chapter 2 discusses the JCAHO's sedation- and anesthesia-related standards in more detail, providing all the compliance information you'll need, and includes tables that identify relevant standards by number.

Chapter 3 addresses credentialing and privileging in the context of sedation and anesthesia care, including an overview of the requirements of the JCAHO and of professional organizations that certify anesthesia providers.

Chapter 4 discusses preparation for a JCAHO survey on the anesthesia standards, concluding with a case study on how St. Joseph's Hospital and Medical Center in Phoenix, Arizona, implemented changes in its anesthesia practice to satisfy JCAHO requirements.

Chapter 5 explains how to develop a quality monitoring program for anesthesia that is based on the continuous quality improvement (CQI) model.

The appendices include a sample moderate ("conscious") sedation policy, sample consent forms, guidelines from the American Society of Anesthesiologists, as well as material to help you educate patients and their families about anesthesia care.

This publication is designed to help you promote safe and effective use of anesthesia, analgesia, and sedation, while also preparing your facility for key elements of its next JCAHO survey.

Anesthesia and Sedation

A focus on improving patient safety in anesthesia care—which began in earnest in the early 1980s with endeavors such as the Anesthesia Patient Safety Foundation—has made administration of anesthetics, sedatives, and analgesics one of the safest high-risk procedures in medicine. Furthermore, with the exception of the administration of conscious sedation, compliance with the JCAHO's standards for anesthetic care has traditionally been among the least troubling accreditation issues. The term *conscious sedation* was problematic in that it required facilities to clearly define the point at which a patient lost "protective reflexes"; and since this was not always obvious, applying anesthesia standards in cases involving conscious sedation has caused considerable confusion for healthcare organizations.

The new JCAHO standards, which include definitions for three levels of sedation (two of which will now trigger both the sedation and the anesthesia standards) as well as anesthesia, should help clarify expectations for care and performance at your next survey. These standards were drafted based on definitions and terminology in "Continuum of Depth of Sedation, Definition of General Anesthesia, and Levels of Sedation/Analgesia," which was approved by the House of Delegates of the American Society of Anesthesiologists on October 13, 1999 (see pp. 140-141). Though the term *moderate sedation* is now preferred, given historical trends, past confusion regarding the term *conscious sedation,* and the implementation of new standards, questions about conscious sedation are likely to come up during your next survey.

A poll of 93 hospitals surveyed during the first three quarters of 1998 revealed the following:

- Surveyors asked about conscious sedation policies during 58% of the surveys.
- They asked about conscious sedation privileges in 48% of the surveys.
- They asked about preoperative assessments 47% of the time.[1]

Finally, 16 hospitals that underwent a JCAHO survey in the first quarter of 1999 reported the following:

- JCAHO surveyors asked 69% of them about their policies on conscious sedation.
- They asked 63% of respondents to identify who in the organization is allowed to administer conscious sedation.
- Surveyors asked 44% of the hospitals to tell them who performs preoperative assessments.
- They asked 56% of the hospitals about anesthesia preassessments.[2]

This book will prepare your organization to respond to such questions, and it will help you design policies and procedures for sedation and anesthesia that improve patient safety and satisfy the expectations of JCAHO surveyors.

---

[1] *Opus Communications, "What's happening during Joint Commission Surveys: Third quarter 1998," A special report from: Briefings on JCAHO, October 1999.*
[2] *Opus Communications, "What's happening during Joint Commission surveys: First quarter 1999," A special report from: Briefings on JCAHO, April 1999.*

When do the JCAHO standards on sedation and anesthesia apply?

Physicians and employees at some facilities believe that the delineated clinical privileges of the practitioner administering conscious sedation determine whether the sedation and anesthesia standards apply. Others think the determining factor is the type of drug(s) in use. These are common misconceptions. In the introduction to the new anesthesia standards, the JCAHO clarifies that "the standards for sedation and anesthesia apply when patients receive, in any setting, for any purpose, by any route, moderate or deep sedation as well as general, spinal, or other major regional anesthesia" (*Comprehensive Accreditation Manual for Hospitals [CAMH]*, August 2000 update, TX-15). According to the JCAHO definition, **moderate sedation is the same as conscious sedation** and is "a drug-induced depression of consciousness during which patients respond purposefully to verbal commands, either alone or accompanied by light tactile stimulation. No interventions are required to maintain a patent airway, and spontaneous ventilation is adequate. Cardiovascular function is usually maintained" (*CAMH*, August 2000 update, TX-15).

The standards will not apply to patients receiving "minimal sedation" or anxiolysis, defined as "a drug-induced state during which patients respond normally to verbal commands. Although cognitive function and coordination may be impaired, ventilation and cardiovascular function is unaffected" (*CAMH*, August 2000 update, TX-15). The process of differentiation between minimal and moderate sedation will present a new challenge to healthcare organizations. For example, they may choose to limit minimal sedation to oral (or in some cases rectal) medications in limited dosages, delegating all parenteral medications to moderate sedation. It is likely JCAHO surveyors will look carefully at the organization's distinction between minimal and

FIGURE 1.1

WHY USE SEDATION?

Frequently, patients who receive one of the three levels of sedation for a procedure will recover more quickly and have fewer side effects, such as nausea and vomiting, than they would have had if they had received a general anesthetic. Sedation is especially preferable for many operative procedures that take place in ambulatory settings and for diagnostic and therapeutic procedures, including

- biopsies,
- laceration repairs,
- orthopedic or podiatric procedures,
- dental or oral surgery procedures,
- gastrointestinal endoscopies,
- bronchoscopies,
- radiographic studies, and
- cardiac catheterizations.

Sedatives and analgesics make it easier for practitioners to complete procedures because they alleviate a patient's pain and anxiety, thus minimizing movement that might compromise the procedure. Practitioners may prefer sedation to anesthesia when they need patients to respond to verbal or tactile stimulation during a procedure. Additionally, unlike anesthesia, in most cases involving sedatives and analgesics, patients are able to interact with the practitioner and to function, as needed, during a procedure.

moderate sedation to assure that patients who experience a "drug-induced depression of consciousness" (moderate sedation) are not cared for as if minimal sedation had been used.

Sedation, which can be administered at different levels of depth, may be preferred to anesthesia for a variety of procedures and patients (see Figure 1.1, p. 4). It is important that institutions and their practitioners clearly evaluate and define situations wherein moderate or deep sedation should be used to ensure that JCAHO standards are met.

Key requirements of the JCAHO standards

Chapter 2 examines all the JCAHO standards relevant to sedation and anesthesia care. However, a few of those standards are particularly relevant to this chapter's discussion.

Patient assessments

Standards in the "Care of Patients (TX)" chapter of the *CAMH* and in the chapter titled "Assessment of Patients (PE)" require hospitals to evaluate all patients before they undergo a procedure involving moderate or deep sedation or anesthesia—an evaluation that is known as a "presedation" or "preanesthetic" assessment. From an accreditation standpoint, the implications of this requirement clearly illustrate why organizations must have criteria for distinguishing between minimal sedation (anxiolysis), moderate sedation (formerly referred to as conscious sedation), and deep sedation. Additionally, because sedation is a continuum and it is not always possible to predict the response a patient will have to medications, practitioners and facilities should be prepared to care for patients if they should enter a deeper level of sedation. For example, patients receiving moderate sedation may enter deep sedation. Likewise, patients receiving deep sedation may enter general anesthesia. Practitioners must be prepared to "rescue" patients from these situations, and sufficient numbers of qualified personnel and equipment must be available to provide the evaluation, monitoring, and care after the procedure.

Clearly, it is impossible for physicians and other practitioners to predict every instance in which patients may enter a deeper level of sedation. Many variables come into play, including

- the patient's age and health status;
- the drug dosage and method of administration;
- the additive effects of sedatives and/or analgesics used in combination; and
- the additive effects of other drugs the patient is taking.

The more data-driven your criteria for assessing sedation cases, the better off you're likely to be during a JCAHO survey. The JCAHO's performance improvement (PI) standards list medication use—which includes use of sedatives, analgesics, and anesthetics—among the six high-risk, high-volume, problem-prone processes that hospitals must monitor (*CAMH,* August 2000 update, PI.3.1.1). Since several variables affect the way patients respond to sedatives and analgesics, and because reactions to these medications can be severe, organizations should consider tracking and evaluating instances when patients receiving sedation enter a deeper level of sedation—for example, when a moderate sedation becomes a deep sedation or a deep sedation becomes general anesthesia. The data might make administration of sedation safer (a key goal of the JCAHO's anesthesia standards) by identifying trends that help you hone your assessment criteria for sedation patients.

Comparable levels of care

A key standard in the "Leadership (LD)" chapter of the *CAMH* requires organizations to provide patients with a comparable level of care—regardless of the treatment setting, and no matter who provides that care. In the context of this chapter, this requirement means organizations must subject practitioners to the same policies, procedures, and standards of care for sedation regardless of whether those practitioners provide the services in an inpatient operating room, an ambulatory surgical center, an examination room, or anywhere else within an organization's facilities. This has become an increasingly important requirement since the changing economics of healthcare began to trigger a wave of facility mergers and the development of multisetting health systems— trends that have increased the range of treatment settings that exist within many organizations.

Given this mandate for a comparable level of care, organizations that are designing a performance improvement program for sedation and anesthesia should consider tracking adverse sedation outcomes by treatment setting and practitioner type. To maximize patient safety and satisfy the JCAHO surveyors, organizations need to ensure that all practitioners who are allowed to administer sedatives, analgesics, and anesthetics do so with equal skill and precision— whether they are anesthesiologists, other physicians with appropriate privileges, or certified registered nurse anesthetists (CRNAs). If performance data reveals quality gaps among practitioner types, or if it suggests that quality varies according to the treatment setting, the organization may need to revise its privileging criteria (see Chapter 3) and sedation policies.

Compliance basics

The JCAHO's *Comprehensive Accreditation Manual for Hospitals (CAMH)* outlines hundreds of standards, all of which serve as fodder for surveyor questions. Given that, it's easy to see how organizations get bogged down in minutiae as they prepare for a survey. However, it's possible to focus so closely on details that you ignore the broader intent of the JCAHO standards:

> The standards are simply articulations of the expectation that organizations will do the "right things right." And when that happens, the likelihood of bad outcomes is minimized and the potential for good outcomes is optimized (*CAMH*, February 1998 update, FW-1).

It's often more useful and effective to prepare for a JCAHO survey by stepping back from the standards and asking everyone in the organization to answer one basic question: If I were the patient, what would I want from the person performing my job? We'll examine this question as it pertains to sedation in Chapter 2, but for now it's worth noting that answers you'll receive usually generate a list of objectives similar to those laid out in the JCAHO standards. If organizations can honestly say their written policies and procedures promote a level of treatment consistent with those objectives, and if they have data documenting that performance and quality of care consistently meet those objectives, they're likely to satisfy the JCAHO.

That said, healthcare organizations should take some basic steps to demonstrate to surveyors that whenever patients receive moderate or deep sedation or anesthesia, the standards and intents for this care are met. Patients receiving minimal sedation (anxiolysis) do not require the care defined in the anesthesia and sedation standards. But verbiage in the JCAHO standards clearly states that patients receiving minimal sedation "respond normally to verbal commands" and do not experience the "drug-induced depression of consciousness" of moderate sedation.

Remember: The nature of the procedure, the classification of drug(s) used, and the qualifications or privileges of the practitioner administering those drugs do not determine when the sedation and anesthesia standards apply. Rather, it is the differentiation between minimal sedation (anxiolysis) and moderate ("conscious") sedation that is the determinant.

The JCAHO's New Sedation- and Anesthesia- Related Standards

The new JCAHO standards for sedation and anesthesia, as set forth in the *CAMH,* apply "when patients receive, in any setting, for any purpose, by any route, moderate or deep sedation as well as general, spinal, or other major regional anesthesia" (*CAMH,* August 2000 update, TX-15). The new standards incorporate the following definitions of four levels of sedation and anesthesia outlined in ASA's "Continuum of Depth of Sedation, Definition of General Anesthesia, and Levels of Sedation/Analgesia" (see pp. 140-141).

1. Minimal sedation (anxiolysis)

A drug-induced state during which patients respond normally to verbal commands. Although cognitive function and coordination may be impaired, ventilatory and cardiovascular functions are unaffected.

2. Moderate sedation/analgesia ("conscious sedation")

A drug-induced depression of consciousness during which patients respond purposefully to verbal commands, either alone or accompanied by light tactile stimulation. No interventions are required to maintain a patent airway, and spontaneous ventilation is adequate. Cardiovascular function is usually maintained.

3. Deep sedation/analgesia

A drug-induced depression of consciousness during which patients cannot be easily aroused but respond purposefully following repeated or painful stimulation. The ability to independently maintain ventilatory function may be impaired. Patients may require assistance in maintaining a patent airway, and spontaneous ventilation may be inadequate. Cardiovascular function is usually maintained.

4. Anesthesia

Consists of general anesthesia and spinal or major regional anesthesia. It does not include local anesthesia. General anesthesia is the drug-induced loss of consciousness during which patients are not arousable, even by painful stimulation. The ability to independently maintain ventilatory function is often impaired. Patients often require assistance in maintaining a patent airway, and positive pressure ventilation may be required because of depressed spontaneous ventilation or drug-induced depression of neuromuscular function. Cardiovascular function may be impaired.

The link between safety, quality, and compliance

Complying with JCAHO standards and maintaining JCAHO accreditation can be challenging, time consuming, and frustrating. It is not uncommon to hear members of hospital and medical staffs complain that the time they spend dealing with compliance issues and survey preparation takes away from their top priority: caring for patients. In some instances they're just blowing off steam, but in others they've lost sight of an important fact: The JCAHO standards are designed to promote safe, effective patient care. Viewed in this light, compliance might not become less arduous, but it will come to seem less like an irrelevant distraction. This view can also form the foundation for a powerful and effective approach to survey preparation.

Pretend you are the patient

Once organizations begin to view the JCAHO standards as a vehicle for maintaining and improving quality of care and patient safety, they're likely to spend less time reading the fine print in their JCAHO standards manual and more time talking about what's best for patients. Survey coordinators and hospital and physician leaders can lead this shift by focusing survey preparation on a basic question: "If each of you were being treated here, what would you want from this organization and its caregivers?"

To assess compliance with the sedation and anesthesia standards, an organization's survey coordinator should ask leaders from anesthesiology a version of the same question: "If you were admitted to this hospital for an operation or some other procedure that involves anesthesia or sedation, what would you expect of the people responsible for that anesthesia or sedation?" The answers usually sound something like this:

- Pick the safest, most effective anesthetics or sedatives.
- Know how to administer them properly.
- Know the contraindications and side effects associated with those medications.
- Learn something about my past experiences with anesthesia or sedation ahead of time.
- Tell me what to expect.
- Allow me ample opportunity to ask questions.
- Answer my questions honestly and with authority.
- Know how I'm doing at all times during the procedure.
- Don't rush off to the next patient and procedure before making sure the practitioners and nurses monitoring my recovery have the information they need to do a good job.
- Do all of the above whether I'm to be sedated or anesthetized.

Once you've brainstormed as many responses as possible, compare your answers with the compliance requirements discussed in the section that follows. You'll probably find that you have addressed most of the major issues. Next, ask yourselves whether your current policies, procedures, and treatment systems are consistent with the responses you generated, and ask whether your staff implement those policies, procedures, and systems effectively. If the answer to both questions is yes, you should be in good survey shape. Furthermore, if JCAHO surveyors think otherwise, you should have solid grounds for appealing Type I recommendations. If the answer to either question is no, use your responses and the guidance provided in this chapter to make the necessary changes to your policies, procedures, and systems.

What standards apply to anesthesia care?

The JCAHO standards governing sedation and anesthesia are designed to protect patient safety and promote quality care in all settings where patients receive anesthetics, sedatives, and/or analgesics. The largest concentration of standards related to sedation and anesthesia care occurs in the chapter titled Care of Patients (TX) in the JCAHO's *Comprehensive Accreditation Manual for Hospitals (CAMH)*—specifically, standards TX.2 through TX.2.4.1. However, healthcare facilities will also find standards that have direct or indirect implications for anesthesia care in the following *CAMH* chapters:

- Patient Rights and Organization Ethics (RI)
- Assessment of Patients (PE)
- Patient and Family Education (PF)
- Continuum of Care (CC)

- Improving Organization Performance (PI)
- Leadership (LD)
- Management of the Environment of Care (EC)
- Management of Human Resources (HR)
- Management of Information (IM)
- Surveillance, Prevention, and Control of Infection (IC)
- Medical Staff (MS)

Because the JCAHO includes relevant standards in so many *CAMH* chapters, some hospitals find it difficult to educate caregivers and monitor compliance. This chapter is meant to assist them by providing a comprehensive overview of the JCAHO's requirements.

The sedation and anesthesia standards and tips on compliance

Having adequate policy and procedure documents in place is only half the battle during a JCAHO survey. During interview sessions and visits to patient care areas, surveyors will question hospital staff and physicians to gauge how effectively they implement and understand the hospital's policies, procedures, and standards of care. The following list should give you a taste of the questions surveyors might ask:

- What are your criteria for determining appropriate levels of sedation for patients undergoing diagnostic or therapeutic procedures?
- How do you assess patients before they receive moderate or deep sedation or anesthesia? Who assesses these patients?

- Where and when do practitioners responsible for administering sedation or anesthesia meet their patients?
- How does the facility coordinate anesthesia services with surgical and nursing services?
- Is anesthesia or sedation ever administered outside the operating room? Where?
- Who monitors patients receiving anesthesia and sedation outside the operating room? How is that monitoring accomplished?
- What are the criteria for discharging patients from the postanesthesia care unit?
- Does your facility track adverse events and outcomes in patients receiving anesthesia and sedation?
- How do you ensure that only qualified practitioners administer or supervise anesthesia and sedation?

The following sections should help you prepare hospital staff and physicians to answer these and other questions by explaining the JCAHO's standards and offering compliance advice. Each section begins with a list of the relevant standards that will be addressed in that section (note that specific standard numbers are subject to periodic change). To avoid repetition and to promote a multidisciplinary approach to anesthesia care, there is not a section for each standard—nor are the sections organized by *CAMH* chapter. This discussion addresses the goals, expectations, and themes that run throughout the standards and across different *CAMH* chapters. Facilities where policies, procedures, and caregiver performance are consistent with the treatment objectives and activities discussed here should be well prepared for a JCAHO survey.

Informed consent for anesthesia and sedation

RELEVANT STANDARDS

RI.1.1–RI.1.2.7

TX 2.2

TX.5.2–TX.5.2.2

An important aspect of providing quality care involves ensuring that patients understand and agree to the care they receive. JCAHO standards require that the healthcare organization and physician(s) document that they have informed patients and obtained consent prior to any invasive or other high-risk procedure. This expectation applies to

- operative procedures;
- the administration of anesthesia or sedation in doses that may cause patients to lose their ability to maintain independent ventilatory function (moderate or deep sedation); or
- the administration of blood or blood products.

Informed consent involves more than a signature on a consent form. The treating physician must also discuss the procedure or treatment with the patient, and allow ample opportunity for the patient and family to ask questions. Important elements of this dialogue include

- a description of the procedure in terms easily understood by the patient;
- the potential risks and benefits;

- potential problems following the treatment or procedure;
- potential for success (or failure);
- consequences of not performing the treatment or procedure; and
- any alternatives to the treatment or procedure.

The treating physician must provide written documentation of this discussion in the preoperative evaluation, history and physical, progress notes, or as a part of the patient consent form.

In situations where the patient is unable to directly offer informed consent (e.g., the patient is a minor or an adult who has been deemed unable to make such decisions), a surrogate decision-maker, such as a parent or other relative, a guardian, or an authorized acquaintance may provide informed consent. The JCAHO defines *surrogate decision-maker* as "someone appointed to act on behalf of another . . . when an individual is without capacity or has given permission to involve others" (*CAMH*, August 1998 update, GL-24).

Facilities, physicians, and other caregivers must also respect and protect the rights of patients participating in clinical studies. They must ensure that these patients have been informed of the potential benefits, risks, and alternatives to participation and that they take part in the study willingly. Patients must fully understand any procedure, including sedation or anesthesia if it is utilized. Healthcare facilities must have a written policy outlining acceptable procedures for informing patients and securing consent, and practitioners must document these efforts.

A consent form frequently provides documentation that the patient understands and agrees to proceed with a specific treatment or procedure. However, as stated previously, a signed consent form cannot replace the process of informed consent, which includes a discussion between patient and physician. Depending upon the nature of the procedure, the organization's scope of service, or the specialty of the licensed independent practitioner, the consent forms may be combined into single documents or used as separate forms (see pp. 132-138).

The licensed independent practitioner obtaining the informed consent will vary depending upon the procedure. For example, when a laparotomy is performed, the surgeon will obtain consent for the operative procedure while an anesthesiologist will obtain consent for the administration of anesthesia. If blood may be needed, either or both of the physicians may obtain consent. If a brochoscopy is to be performed under moderate sedation by a pulmonologist, the pulmonologist will obtain consent for both the procedure and the moderate sedation.

A patient who has had a "do not resuscitate" (DNR) order written presents special challenges to the healthcare team. Facilities and physicians should ensure that the patient with a DNR order (as well as the patient's family) has had discussions with both the anesthesia care provider and surgeon or other physician performing a procedure. The details of these conversations should be noted in the patient's medical record. Because of potential depression of ventilatory and cardiovascular function under moderate or deep sedation or anesthesia, the physician(s) should inform the patient and family that the DNR order will be rescinded during the treatment or procedure.

■◆ *Compliance Tips*

The following should be helpful hints in obtaining informed consent:

- Obtain informed consent as early as possible during the encounter.
- Discuss alternatives to moderate or deep sedation (e.g., regional, monitored anesthesia care; or general anesthesia, if applicable) as well as the risks and benefits of each.
- Explain the treatment or procedure in terms easily understood by the patient or family.
- Make appropriate accommodations for patients who do not speak English, or who are visually or hearing impaired, such as having interpreters or other qualified individuals available.
- Conduct the informed consent discussion in a comfortable, relaxed environment.
- Include family members in the discussion.
- Allow ample opportunity for the patient and family to engage in an open discussion, with plenty of time for questions and answers.
- Accurately record all conversations in the medical record.
- If an emergency exists and it is not possible to obtain informed consent, practitioners can provide care but must document the situation by clearly describing the situation in the patient record.

Preanesthetic assessments and anesthesia planning

RELEVANT STANDARDS
LD.1.3.4
LD.1.6
MS.6.2.1
PE.1.6–PE.1.6.1.1
PE.1.8–PE.1.8.4
TX.1 & TX.1.2
TX.2–TX.2.4.1
TX.5–TX.5.1.5
TX.5.3

Because anesthesia and sedation place patients at considerable risk—
and because patients may respond differently to anesthetics, sedatives,
and analgesics—careful planning is a key part of quality anesthesia care.
Preanesthesia assessments are an important part of that planning process,
and the JCAHO requires them for all procedures involving moderate
or deep sedation and anesthesia.[1] (Remember: The JCAHO's standards
for sedation and anesthesia include moderate "conscious" sedation,
which is defined as a drug-induced depression of consciousness, deep
sedation, and general or major regional anesthesia.) These assessments help
practitioners to

---

[1] *In an emergency, when there is no time to perform and document a history and physical examination, the JCAHO requires only that the patient's record include a description of the circumstances and the practitioner's preoperative diagnosis.*

- select the most effective drug or combination of drugs with which to anesthetize or sedate patients;
- plan the administration of anesthetics or sedatives;
- administer those drugs safely; and
- interpret data obtained during patient monitoring.

An effective preanesthetic assessment reduces the chances of morbidity or mortality caused by complications from anesthesia or sedation. It should include the following elements:

- an assessment of the patient's potential to slip to a deeper level of sedation, and a plan for how the practitioner would react to such a situation;
- an interview with the patient and/or the patient's legal guardian or surrogate decision-maker, which includes a review of the patient's medical history and a focused physical examination [2] (see Figure 2.1); and
- orders for diagnostic tests, including blood work, radiographic studies, an electrocardiogram, and pulmonary functions studies—if the history and physical examination suggest they are necessary. Results of these tests must appear in the patient's medical record.

JCAHO surveyors will assess your compliance with assessment requirements by interviewing physicians and other relevant caregivers, as well as by reviewing a sample of medical records for patients who received anesthesia and/or sedation. The practitioner who administers the anesthesia or sedation does not have to be the one who records notes on the preanesthetic assessment

---

[2] *If a practitioner performed a history and physical examination (H&P) on the patient within 30 days of the patient's date of admission, that H&P may be used during the preanesthetic assessment, "provided durable, legible copies (or originals) of the report are in the patient's record and any significant changes in the patient's condition since the report are recorded at the time of admission" (CAMH, PE.1.5).*

FIGURE 2.1

HISTORY & PHYSICAL CHECKLIST

Medical history:

- ❏ Past medical illness and surgical procedures
- ❏ Drug history, including medication allergies, routine prescription and nonprescription medication use
- ❏ Past anesthetics, including problems or complications with medications, past anesthetics, or procedures in the patient or family
- ❏ History of tobacco or alcohol use, and abuse of controlled or illegal substances
- ❏ History of adverse symptoms related to the patient's daily activity or physical exertion (cardiovascular, respiratory, and neurologic systems) must be investigated and recorded
- ❏ Specific syndromes or associated congenital anomalies
- ❏ Family history of problems with anesthesia, such as malignant hyperthermia

Focused physical examination:

- ❏ Results of all appropriate diagnostic tests
- ❏ Assessment of the patient's physical, mental, and neurological status
- ❏ Vital signs, including heart rate, respiratory rate, blood pressure, and temperature
- ❏ Evaluation of teeth, jaw, neck, heart, lungs, and central and peripheral nervous system for abnormalities of the airway, cardiorespiratory system, and nervous system

and anesthesia plan in the patient's chart, but that chart should include the following preoperative information:

- the patient's anesthesia classification code (see Figure 2.2), which helps a practitioner identify risks to the patient, appropriate drug(s), monitoring methods, and clinical monitoring parameters;
- the type of sedation or anesthesia care to be delivered: moderate or deep sedation, general, regional, or monitored anesthesia care;[3]
- plans or orders for additional preprocedure diagnostic data, if needed, and the results of diagnostic tests performed to obtain that data;
- a practitioner's preoperative diagnosis; and
- a plan, developed prior to the procedure, for nursing care during and after administration of anesthesia or moderate or deep sedation.

The patient must undergo a second preanesthesia/presedation assessment immediately prior to the administration of the anesthesia or moderate or deep sedation (PE.1.8.3). This reassessment ensures that there have been no changes since the initial assessment and that the patient remains a safe candidate for the planned medication(s). It usually includes an evaluation of the patient's blood pressure, heart rate, respiratory rate, mental status, electrocardiogram, and blood oxygenation by pulse oximetry.

---

[3] *"Monitored anesthesia care is a specific anesthesia service in which an anesthesiologist has been [asked] to participate in the care of a patient undergoing a diagnostic or therapeutic procedure. Monitored anesthesia care includes all aspects of anesthesia care—a preprocedure visit, intraoperative care, and postprocedure management" (American Society of Anesthesiologists 2001 Directory of Members, "Position on Monitored Anesthesia Care," Washington, DC: ASA, 2001). The ASA position statement goes on to say that the services provided during monitored anesthesia care include monitoring of vital signs and airway management, diagnosis and treatment of problems occurring during the procedure, administration of medications to enhance patient comfort and safety, and provision of other services as needed. It acknowledges that monitored anesthesia care refers to clinical situations in which patients may or may not lose consciousness.*

ASA PHYSICAL STATUS CLASSIFICATION

P1—A normal, healthy patient

P2—A patient with mild systemic disease

P3—A patient with severe systemic disease

P4—A patient with severe systemic disease that is a constant threat to life

P5—A moribund patient who is not expected to survive without the operation

P6—A declared brain-dead patient whose organs are being removed for donor purposes

© 1999, American Society of Anesthesiologists, 520 N. Northwest Highway, Park Ridge, IL 60068. Reprinted by permission.

The JCAHO requires hospitals to administer anesthesia for obstetric and emergency surgical services within 30 minutes of the determination by the attending physician that anesthesia is necessary. The JCAHO also requires facilities to provide anesthesia for other procedures within a "reasonable time frame" after the preanesthetic assessment—leaving it up to the organization to decide what constitutes a reasonable time frame.

 Compliance Tips

A facility's written policies and procedures are a key element of compliance with the JCAHO requirements regarding preanesthetic assessments and sedation and anesthesia planning. JCAHO surveyors will expect you to have written documents requiring practitioners to fulfill the minimum requirements for preanesthesia care that are outlined above. Furthermore, they'll expect these policies—and your enforcement of them—to apply equally to all treatment settings within your organization. As was discussed in Chapter 1, JCAHO standards require all practitioners within a single organization to provide a comparable level of care, regardless of the treatment setting. With the development of health systems and networks, organizations commonly have a number of treatment settings where patients receive moderate or deep sedation or anesthesia for procedures, and JCAHO surveyors carefully gauge quality and performance across settings.

Surveyors assess the performance of caregivers and the quality of care provided in your organization in two basic ways: (1) by interviewing physicians and staff and (2) by reviewing caregiver documentation in patient medical records. As you prepare for a survey, ensure that relevant caregivers can describe their roles and responsibilities in preanesthesia care as they are outlined in your policies and procedures. You should also periodically audit chart documentation to ensure that it indicates that practitioners consistently provide safe, high-quality preanesthesia care, as defined by your policies, and that they document the provision of that care clearly and adequately. Because documentation at this stage of anesthesia care is recorded on a number of different documents, your facility should consider creating a checklist to track it all.

Although it is not required by the JCAHO, facilities should consider incorporating relevant elements of the American Society of Anesthesiologists' "Guidelines for Patient Care in Anesthesiology" (see pp. 151-153) and all elements of ASA's "Basic Standards for Preanesthesia Care" (see p. 155) into documents that formalize their policies and procedures for preanesthesia assessment and planning. The guidelines in these ASA documents are consistent with many of the JCAHO's preanesthesia requirements and can help improve the quality and safety of anesthesia care.

Intraoperative anesthesia care

```
RELEVANT STANDARDS
        TX.2.3
        PE.1.8.3
        IM.7.3
        LD.1.3.2
        LD.2.7
        LD.2.9
```

Like patients receiving general anesthesia, sedated patients might lose the ability to communicate, which means physiologic monitoring may be the only means of determining their well-being. Monitoring allows practitioners to evaluate the effects of the medication and the procedure on the patient and to intervene in emergencies such as airway obstruction, bronchospasm, arrythmias, or hypotension.

An authorized practitioner must monitor the heart and respiratory rates, electrocardiogram, blood pressure, and oxygenation of all patients receiving anesthesia or moderate or deep sedation. Whether additional monitoring is necessary depends on the results of the preanesthesia assessment and the final assessment made before the procedure begins; the nature of the procedure; and the anesthetics or sedatives slated for use. All physiological data collected during the procedure must be documented in the patient's medical record.

Organizations should consider incorporating the ASA's "Standards for Basic Anesthetic Monitoring" (see pp. 147-150) into policy and procedure documents that govern intraoperative anesthesia care. In general, these documents should

- outline appropriate monitoring methods and procedures;
- identify criteria for determining which methods and procedures to use; and
- detail minimum requirements regarding documentation of monitoring data (e.g., time intervals for documenting, specificity of documentation, etc.).

 Compliance Tips

As with most standards, JCAHO surveyors assess compliance with intraoperative anesthesia requirements by interviewing physicians and staff, reviewing policy and procedure documents, and auditing medical record documentation. Prior to your next survey, ensure that relevant caregivers understand and can explain their roles and responsibilities during intraoperative anesthesia care. You should also review and, if necessary, revise your policies and procedures to ensure that they address the minimum requirements outlined above. And you should audit a representative sample of medical records to ensure that the anesthesia records in them document the following information for all relevant procedures:

- patient's vital signs at regular, appropriate intervals;
- the dosage of all drugs given and the time of administration;
- all fluids a patient received, including blood and blood products;
- an estimate of the volume of blood and other fluids lost by the patient;
- the method for administering anesthetics, sedatives, and/or analgesics;

- any unusual events or complications; and
- the status of the patient at the conclusion of a procedure involving anesthesia or moderate or deep sedation.

Postanesthesia care

```
            R E L E V A N T   S T A N D A R D S

                         PE.1.8.4

                    TX.2.4 & TX.2.4.1

                         TX.5.4

                         IM.7.3.3

                   IM.7.3.4 & IM.7.3.4.1

                         IM.7.3.5
```

At the end of a procedure involving anesthesia or moderate or deep sedation, patients usually go to a designated postanesthesia care unit (PACU)— although some go to intensive care. In the PACU, a caregiver is assigned to monitor the patient continuously and implement an LIP's orders for postanesthesia care—notifying the appropriate LIP(s) of changes for better or worse in the patient's condition and documenting information regarding

- fluids, including blood or blood products, that the patient received or lost (i.e., the amounts received or lost and the resulting effects);
- medications administered; and
- the patient's physiological and mental status, including
  - blood pressure, heart rate, respiratory rate, and blood oxygenation;
  - body temperature;

- level of consciousness;
- circulation (perfusion of tissues);
- condition of dressings (if relevant);
- types of drains (e.g., chest tube) and the nature and quantity of drainage;
- condition of intravenous site(s) and the type, amount, and effects of solutions (medication, blood and blood products, other fluids) being infused;
- changes in the patient's general appearance (e.g., edema, rashes, etc.);
- diaphoresis (perspiration);
- discomfort, restlessness, or apprehension; and
- complications or unexpected developments.

Depending on the nature of the procedure and the type of anesthesia or sedation used, the PACU caregiver should monitor and document other things—as required by facility policy or ordered by an LIP. Following spinal anesthesia, for example, caregivers monitor and document the patient's ability to move his or her lower extremities.

An LIP must evaluate patients before they leave the PACU, and/or the patients must meet discharge criteria that have been approved by the facility's medical staff. These criteria should include

- stable blood pressure, heart rate, and respiratory rate;
- clearly defined level of consciousness;
- no excessive bleeding; and
- no evidence of other physiological instability.

The medical record must include the name of the LIP responsible for discharging a patient and show that the patient met the facility's discharge criteria. If the patient is sent directly home from the PACU—rather than being transferred to another care setting—he or she must be accompanied by an adult.

 Compliance Tips

Facilities must have a policy that governs patient care during the postanesthesia period. They should consider using ASA's "Standards for Postanesthesia Care" (see pp. 155-157) when developing that policy. Their policy must apply to all patients who receive general anesthesia, major regional anesthesia, or moderate or deep sedation. In general, the policy should require

- PACUs to have specified medical and nursing leadership;
- comparable levels of care in PACUs throughout an organization or facility; and
- compliance with identical discharge criteria in PACUs throughout the organization or facility.

The policy must also outline requirements for monitoring of vital signs and other key indicators, detailing which physiological functions and indicators PACU caregivers must monitor and indicating how frequently they must record their observations in the medical record.

Provider collaboration during anesthesia and sedation

```
┌─────────────────────────────────────────────────────┐
│  ┌───────────────────────────────────────────────┐  │
│  │             RELEVANT STANDARD                 │  │
│  │                                               │  │
│  │                   TX.1.2                      │  │
│  └───────────────────────────────────────────────┘  │
└─────────────────────────────────────────────────────┘
```

To satisfy JCAHO standards and, more importantly, to enhance patient safety and quality of care, planning for and management of anesthesia care must be interdisciplinary. It should involve collaboration among all practitioners involved in a specific procedure or in the general oversight of a patient's care. The treatment team should agree on goals and expectations for administration of and recovery from anesthesia or moderate or deep sedation, and team members should involve the patient and the patient's family in this process whenever possible.

Compliance Tips

A facility can demonstrate that it provides multidisciplinary sedation and anesthesia care—involving nurses, anesthesiologists and/or CRNAs, surgical and medical practitioners, etc.—by reviewing a number of key documents with JCAHO surveyors, including

- written policies and procedures;
- medical records (especially all anesthesia assessments, anesthesia plans; and progress notes); and
- transfer summaries (see Figure 2.3).

FIGURE 2.3

TRANSFER SUMMARY FORM

Transfer Summary

Patient name (last, first, middle) _____

Attending physician _____

Principal diagnosis _____

Secondary diagnosis _____

Date of transfer _____ Record # _____

Transfer vital signs
Pulse _____ Oxygen sat _____ BP _____ Temp _____

Allergies _____

Medications _____
_____

Reason for transfer
❏ Observation for apnea
❏ Other   Explain _____
_____

Transfer nursing assessment
_____
_____

Instructions given to patient's primary caregiver
_____
_____

Signature of nurse _____ Date _____

Adapted from a form provided by Turville Bay MRI Center. Concept used with permission.

Anesthesia, sedation, and the medication use standards

```
┌─────────────────────────────────────────────┐
│  RELEVANT STANDARDS                            │
│                                                │
│              TX.3.3                            │
│                                                │
│              TX.3.4                            │
│                                                │
│              TX.3.5                            │
│                                                │
│              TX.3.5.3                          │
│                                                │
│              TX.3.5.6                          │
│                                                │
│              TX.3.8                            │
│                                                │
│              TX.3.9                            │
└─────────────────────────────────────────────┘
```

Each year when the JCAHO identifies the standards with which hospitals have the most trouble complying, medication use standards routinely rank among the top ten. In 2000, for instance, the standard that addresses security and control of medication ranked as the second most common source of Type I recommendations. Anesthetics, sedatives, and analgesics are, of course, medications—which means that they're subject to both the JCAHO's medication use standards in addition to the anesthesia standards.

Enactment and enforcement of a medication use policy that addresses a number of key issues (see Figure 2.4) is key to compliance. As with the anesthesia standards, the JCAHO's medication use standards are designed to promote patient safety and quality of care. Organizations that design policies and procedures and train physicians and staff with safety and quality in mind are likely to find that they comply with many of the medication use standards.

FIGURE 2.4 **KEY ELEMENTS OF A MEDICATION USE POLICY**

A facility must develop and enforce a policy governing medication use. The policy must be consistent with state and federal law and should describe who is authorized to prescribe and/or administer medications. It should also address

- restrictions on the use of medications under specific conditions or in specific treatment settings;
- requirements for storing and accessing medications when the pharmacy is open and, if relevant, after it has closed for the day;
- procedures for ordering medications;
- guidelines for preparing and administering medications;
- systems for verifying the "five Rs" (right patient, right drug, right dose, right time, and right route of administration) prior to administration;
- requirements for monitoring patients after drug administration;
- procedures for identifying and preventing medication allergies and food-drug or drug-drug interactions;
- procedures, consistent with state and federal law, for storing, distributing, and administering controlled substances;
- requirements for obtaining and documenting the informed consent of patients before administration of investigational drugs;
- development of and compliance with the organization's drug formulary;
- procedures for ordering medications not on the formulary;
- requirements for use of vasoactive drugs (e.g., administration by infusion pump may need to be accompanied by carefully documented invasive blood pressure monitoring); and
- procedures for identifying and reporting adverse drug reactions, medication errors, and other adverse drug events.

What follows is a discussion of the medication use standards that are most relevant to anesthesia care. It addresses the main goals of the medication use standards—controlling access to medications, maintaining the safety and effectiveness of drug treatment, and monitoring outcomes of drug treatment—by focusing on what the JCAHO sees as the five core processes of medication use systems: (1) selection, procurement, and storage; (2) prescribing and ordering; (3) preparation and dispensing; (4) administration; and (5) monitoring effects on the patient (*CAMH*, August 1997 update, TX-20).

Selection, procurement, and storage of medications

The standards that address selection, procurement, and storage of medications call for the creation of a formulary—an inventory of drugs that an organization stocks and allows practitioners to prescribe. The JCAHO expects the development and maintenance of this formulary to be an ongoing, collaborative, and multidisciplinary process that takes into account the needs of an organization's patient population as well as a drug's safety, effectiveness, and cost. However, the JCAHO recognizes that cases may arise in which a patient needs medication not on the formulary, and it expects organizations to establish effective policies and procedures for addressing these cases.

JCAHO surveyors also expect to see evidence that caregivers are familiar with safe and effective methods for storing medications and that an organization takes steps to ensure that drugs are stored properly and securely. The standards do not assign responsibility to any one department for coordinating medication storage and control, but they imply that the pharmacy is probably best prepared to accept it.

Compliance Tips

To comply with the standards related to selection, procurement, and storage of medications, an organization should be prepared to show JCAHO surveyors a written copy of its formulary, along with documentation (e.g., meeting minutes) demonstrating that a multidisciplinary task force—with representatives from the medical, pharmacy, nursing, and administrative staffs—reviews the formulary and considers changes to it. In most hospitals, the pharmacy and therapeutics committee performs these reviews and submits formulary recommendations to the medical executive committee for consideration. An organization should have written policies that govern (1) maintenance of the formulary; (2) procedures for ordering and procuring nonformulary medications; and (3) storage and control of medications. Clinical staff on the formulary-review task force and in patient-care areas should be familiar with these policies.

Prescribing and ordering

The JCAHO requires organizations to institute formal procedures for limiting risks associated with prescribing and ordering medication. The standards identify ten specific areas that organizations need to address, seven of which are relevant to anesthesia and sedation:

1. distribution, administration and/or disposal of controlled medications (such as narcotics and sedatives or hypnotics), including adequate documentation and record keeping, as required by state and federal law;
2. proper storage, distribution, and control of investigational medications and those in clinical trial;

3. situations in which all or some of a patient's medication orders must be permanently or temporarily canceled, and mechanisms for reinstating them;

4. "as needed" (PRN) prescriptions or orders and times of dose administration;

5. control of sample drugs;

6. distribution of medications to patients at discharge; and

7. procurement, storage, control, and distribution of prepackaged medications obtained from outside sources (*CAMH*, August 2000 update, TX.3.3).

Compliance Tips

Organizations need to have policies and procedures for each of the areas listed above. Among other things, they need to be certain that these policies identify who can prescribe and order medications for patients (by law, this is limited to licensed physicians and, in some states, nurse practitioners and physician assistants) and outline guidelines and procedures regarding the maintenance, availability, and use of patient medication profiles (see Figure 2.5).

Since many anesthetics, sedatives, and analgesics are controlled substances, it is worth highlighting requirements regarding the handling and disposal of controlled substances. State and federal laws addressing this topic are strict. For instance, if a patient does not receive the full contents of a container holding a controlled substance, a licensed caregiver must witness the disposal of the leftover portion. In addition, the facility must document the disposal procedures, the name of the person handling the disposal, and the name of the witness. Most facilities develop adequate policies and procedures for handling controlled substances, but many receive Type I recommendations for failing to comply consistently and/or in all treatment settings with those policies and procedures.

FIGURE 2.5

THE PATIENT MEDICATION PROFILE

The patient medication profile (PMP) contains the specific information on a patient's condition, medical history, and medication treatment regimen that caregivers need to ensure the safety of that patient during drug treatment. Every patient who takes medication must have a PMP, and the PMP should be available to and easily accessed by pharmacy staff, nurses, and physicians. All staff involved in patient care should be able to add notations to the PMP, but only a pharmacist should have the authority and ability to change information in a PMP. Ideally, organizations make the PMP available by computer, which facilitates access and may allow more than one person to refer to a patient's profile simultaneously.

Following is a list of information that should generally appear in the PMP:

- the patient's name, birthdate, and gender;
- the patient's current height and weight;
- the patient's problems, symptoms, and/or diagnoses;
- all current medications a patient is taking—including investigational drugs;
- all known allergies and medication sensitivities;
- potential food-drug and/or drug-drug interactions;
- information, if relevant, on a patient's use of illegal drugs;
- information, if relevant, on a patient's misuse of prescription drugs;
- creatinine and BUN values for patients who are over 65 or candidates for kidney dysfunction; and
- body-surface area for chemotherapy patients.

As with all patient information, organizations should take steps to protect the confidentiality of medication profiles.

Preparation and dispensing

These standards apply most directly to pharmacy practices. JCAHO expects organizations to comply with all laws, regulations, and practice standards governing the preparation and dispensing of medications and the licensing of individuals who prepare and dispense drugs. Surveyors will also want to see evidence that organizations

- employ standardized dosing, distribution, and labeling procedures to help prevent medication errors;
- have procedures for preventing patients from receiving expired medications; and
- have pharmacists review all prescriptions and medication orders— except in specific clinical and emergency situations, as outlined in the standards manual (*CAMH*, August 2000 update, TX.3.5.2).

The JCAHO insists that diagnoses, known allergies, and other patient information be available to support reviews of prescriptions and orders and help individuals involved in preparing and dispensing medication to

- facilitate continuity of care;
- create an accurate medication history;
- supplement monitoring of adverse drug events; and
- provide safe administration of medications (*CAMH*, August 2000 update, TX.3.3).

Finally, the JCAHO expects organizations to have effective procedures in place for tracking dispensed medications—including samples—in case of a discontinuation or recall.

Compliance Tips

To comply with standards governing preparation and dispensing of drugs, the JCAHO recommends that, among other things, hospitals employ a unit-dose drug distribution system. Most organizations do so, but they also should have written policies and procedures to support and facilitate that system, as well as to

- define who has the authority to prepare and dispense medication;
- outline standardized procedures for labeling medication in all preparation areas, including satellite pharmacies;
- mandate that a pharmacist review and initial orders and prescriptions (the policy should also define the scope of these reviews);
- describe the information that must be noted in a patient's chart and medication profile in order to facilitate pharmacist reviews; and
- explain procedures for inspecting drug stocks to ensure that patients do not receive expired, recalled, or discontinued medications.

Hospitals should keep copies of relevant policies, laws, and regulations in the pharmacy and in other areas where medication is prepared and dispensed. They should address this information and accepted standards of practice during training and inservice sessions for staff who are authorized to prepare and dispense medications, and they should document the attendance and the information covered at these sessions.

Organizations should periodically inspect a sampling of medication orders and patient charts to confirm that staff are complying with relevant policies, and they should ensure that the orders are supported by appropriate chart documentation. Those inspections should be documented in writing, and inspection reports should be presented as evidence of compliance during a JCAHO survey.

Administration

The standards that apply to medication administration primarily affect the nursing and medical staffs. They are designed to ensure that properly trained and licensed individuals administer medications to patients, that those people verify orders and patient identification before administering drugs, and that they take other steps to augment the safety and effectiveness of drug treatment. In addition to general medication use, these standards address procedures and policies for dealing with investigational medications and medications that patients bring with them to a hospital.

 Compliance Tips

These standards address what are sometimes called the "five rights" of medication use: right patient, right drug, right dose, right time, and right route of administration. Organizations should have written policies mandating verification of this information and requiring staff to document verification. They should also design and document training and inservice sessions to support these policies. Hospitals might want to consider employing bar coding and other technologies to support and improve the accuracy of verification and identification activities.

Beyond verification activities, these standards require hospitals to design "alternative medication administration systems" for medications that patients bring with them to a hospital and/or that they will be administering to themselves.

If, upon admission to a hospital, patients are on medication, the organization should have procedures in place for factoring that existing regimen into all decisions regarding additional medication use. A physician must assess all medications that patients bring with them to the facility—to determine whether use of the drugs is medically appropriate. If patients bring controlled substances or prescription medications to the hospital, the hospital must confirm that written orders authorized use of the drugs; organizations should have a written policy requiring this confirmation. If patients will be self-administering medications, the organization should have written policies that outline procedures for ensuring that patients understand how to administer their medications and for supporting safe, effective self-administration.

Pain management is another issue that is worth discussing in the context of administration of medications and surveillance of medication use. Many hospitals have developed pain management programs that seek to enhance the comfort of patients—often by allowing nurses to administer pain medication on an as-needed basis or by giving patients the means to self-administer it. Anesthesiologists should coordinate these programs, and for the sake of patient safety and quality of care, facilities should control and monitor them as intensely as they control and monitor medication use in any other setting or situation. Lack of appropriate policies and procedures governing pain management programs frequently results in Type I recommendations during JCAHO surveys.

Monitoring the effects of medication on patients

The current standard that requires organizations to assess the effects of medication on patients is designed to ensure that monitoring activities are interdisciplinary, interactive, and continuous. They require physicians, pharmacists, and nurses to work together to monitor effects, to rely on information in medical records and patient medication profiles, and to seek input from patients and their families.

Compliance Tips

All monitoring activities must be documented in patient medical records, and organizations should have written policies and procedures that address JCAHO requirements governing drug-effects monitoring. As an example, in the context of anesthesia care, hospitals should consider drafting a policy on dealing with malignant hyperthermia, a serious adverse reaction to anesthesia that can cause a patient's body temperature to rise to potentially fatal levels.

An organization's policies should mandate collaboration between physicians, nurses, and pharmacists; should create channels that facilitate and guide this collaboration; and should require caregivers to seek patient input. Among other things, hospital policies and procedures should provide the means for

- pharmacists to question medication orders that seem inconsistent with aspects of patient diagnoses and/or medication profiles;
- nurses to question abnormal doses or pharmacy deliveries that seem inconsistent with medication orders; and
- nurses, physicians, or pharmacists to report the effects of drug treatment, including unexpected outcomes and adverse drug events.

Educating patients and families about anesthesia and sedation

RELEVANT STANDARDS
PF.1 & PF.1.1
PF.1.3
PF.1.5
PF.1.8
PF.3
PF.4.1 & PF.4.2

Patient involvement and cooperation are widely viewed as critical to effective medical treatment. For that reason, the JCAHO has long viewed patient and family education as a cornerstone responsibility of hospitals and caregivers. Informed patients, guardians, and surrogate decision-makers are likely to be more compliant with the treatment plan proposed by caregivers. In addition, they may feel less anxious about high-risk procedures like anesthesia and sedation. Effective methods for educating patients and families about anesthesia and sedation—methods that are tailored to each patient's needs and limitations— play an important role in successful outcomes.

Educating patients, family members, and/or surrogate decision-makers about anesthesia or sedation means explaining

- the benefits and desired outcome;
- the likelihood that the procedure involving anesthesia or sedation will be successful;
- the risks and possible complications;

- alternative approaches to treatment; and
- the likely effect of postponing or canceling the procedures that call for anesthesia or sedation.

Effective education involves finding ways to overcome language barriers and physical or mental disabilities.

 Compliance Tips

Organizations should have a policy that outlines procedures and requirements for educating patients and families. They also must ensure that caregivers document the education they provide.

It is important for caregivers to determine whether individuals are prepared or able to process information about anesthesia care, and to identify the best methods for educating them. To this end, facilities should consider developing assessment forms that will help caregivers identify the educational needs and limitations of patients, family members, and surrogate decision-makers, including

- cultural and/or religious preferences;
- literacy and education levels;
- native language(s);
- relevant disabilities (e.g., deafness, dementia, etc.); and
- emotional state.

Be sure these forms have enough space to note unique desires, needs, or limitations not covered in enough detail elsewhere (see Figures 2.6a and 2.6b). Also, make sure your facility provides caregivers with the necessary educational resources by offering them access to translators, videotapes, audiotapes, written materials (see Appendix C, p. 163), and other materials that will help them respond to the needs of patients, families, and other decision-makers.

Possible food-drug and drug-drug interactions should be a key element of your educational curriculum for anesthesia care. Patients need to understand the risks of such interactions and take steps to help prevent them (e.g., not eating for several hours before a procedure involving anesthesia, telling a practitioner if they have eaten too recently, accurately identifying medications taken before a procedure, etc.). Effective education and communication can help practitioners identify the potential for dangerous interactions, allowing them to modify the sedation or anesthesia plan or to delay sedation or anesthesia until it can be administered safely.

In addition to assessment forms, facilities should consider developing a preoperative program that is designed to teach patients and families basic information about sedation and anesthesia. The program might include a brief presentation, during which caregivers

- explain what will happen before, during, and after anesthesia or sedation; and
- use educational tools (handouts, audiotapes, videos, etc.) to describe the qualifications and roles of caregivers involved in the administration of anesthesia and sedation.

FIGURE 2.6a

INITIAL EDUCATIONAL LEARNING ASSESSMENT

Information source Self _____ Spouse _____ Parent _____ Other, specify: _____

Pre-hospital teaching: Did you participate in any pre-hospital education?
❏ No ❏ Yes, describe: _____

Religious/Cultural practices: Do you have any beliefs or values that we should consider in providing care or education?
❏ No ❏ Yes, describe: _____

Language/Cognition: Language spoken: ❏ English ❏ Other, specify: _____
Educational background: ❏ Grade school ❏ High school ❏ Technical
❏ College ❏ Other, specify: _____

Does you learn best by: ❏ Visualizing ❏ Hearing (Auditory) ❏ Doing (Psychometer)

Is patient's hearing, vision, or speech impaired?
❏ No ❏ Yes, describe: _____ (*Speech)

Can patient follow and understand directions? ❏ Yes ❏ No, describe: _____

Learning aids needed: ❏ Signer ❏ Interpreter ❏ None

Motivation: Is patient/family highly motivated to learn?
❏ Yes ❏ No, describe: _____

Support/Emotional needs: Do you have any emotional/family/home concerns that need to be addressed during your hospitalization? ❏ No ❏ Yes, describe: _____ (*Social services)

Physical limitations: Do you have any physical limitations that may alter care or limit your learning ability?
❏ Yes ❏ No, describe: _____ (*Physical therapy, Occupational therapy)

FIGURE 2.6a *continued*

INITIAL EDUCATIONAL LEARNING ASSESSMENT

Financial implications: Are there any financial issues or concerns?

❏ No   ❏ Yes, describe: _____ (*Social services)

Educational needs: Do you or your family need information on the following?

❏ Current illness   ❏ Medications   ❏ Diet/Nutrition   ❏ Equipment

❏ Home care   ❏ Restraints/Seclusion   ❏ Community resources   ❏ Access to follow-up care

❏ Rehab techniques   ❏ Personal hygiene/Grooming ❏ Pain management   ❏ Food-drug interaction

❏ None   ❏ Other, describe: _____

Is access to schooling needed? (For school-age and adolescent patients with long periods of hospitalization)

❏ No   ❏ Yes

Did you receive a copy of the Patient Rights Booklet?   ❏ Yes   ❏ No, explain: _____

Do you or your family have any questions?   ❏ No   ❏ Yes, explain: _____

Educational needs by priority (as appropriate):

1. _____

2. _____

3. _____

*Send notification on to service, if appropriate.

_____

Signature   Time   Date

_____

Signature   Time   Date

FIGURE 2.6b — EDUCATIONAL NEEDS AND ABILITIES ASSESSMENT

Speech:　❑ Normal　　❑ Problems: _____

Language(s) spoken:　❑ English　❑ Other(s)

Memory problems:　❑ No　　❑ Yes, describe: _____
　　　　　　Recent: ❑ No　　❑ Yes　　Remote: ❑ No　　❑ Yes

Learning problems:　❑ No　　❑ Yes, describe: _____

Learning style:　❑ Visual　　❑ Auditory　　❑ Touch

Education level: (check the highest level)
　　　　❑ Grade school ❑ High school ❑ College　　❑ Postgraduate

Patient perception of reading skills:　❑ Excellent　　❑ Good　　❑ Poor

What do you know about your healthcare problem? _____

Cultural/Spiritual:
Are there any religious, traditional, ethnic, or cultural practices that need to be part of your care?
❑ No　　❑ Yes, describe: _____

Is there any way the hospital can assist you with your religious practices?
❑ No　　❑ Yes, describe: _____

Pre-hospital teaching: Did you participate in any pre-hospital education?
❑ No　　❑ Yes, describe: _____

How best do you learn new information?
❑ Reading　　❑ Audiotapes　　❑ Return demonstration　❑ Video　　❑ Listening　　❑ Touching

Caregiver assessment:
Is patient/family motivated to learn? ❑ Yes　　❑ No, describe: _____

Is patient/family ready to learn?　❑ Yes　　❑ No, describe: _____

Barriers to learning:
Emotional:　　　　　　　❑ Yes　　❑ No, describe: _____

Physical impairment　　　❑ Yes　　❑ No, describe: _____

Cognitive impairments　　❑ Yes　　❑ No, describe: _____

Is patient beginning to ask questions about disease, treatment, medications, or equipment?
❑ No　　❑ Yes, describe _____

Reprinted by permission of St. Alexius Medical Center, Bismark ND.

Anesthesia, sedation, and the continuum of care

RELEVANT STANDARDS

CC.4

CC.5

CC.6 & CC.6.1

CC.7

It is not unusual for several caregivers to treat a patient over the course
of one or more treatment episodes. For that treatment to be as safe
and effective as possible, the transfer of patient information among
caregivers, treatment settings, and treatment episodes must be efficient
and flawless. The JCAHO's continuum of care (CC) standards require
seamless transitions across treatment settings and among caregivers.

In the context of sedation and anesthesia care, continuity is dependent
on three factors: (1) patient and family education, (2) information management, and (3) practitioner collaboration and communication. If patients,
family members, and surrogate decision-makers are not educated effectively
about anesthesia care, they may not provide the information necessary to
ensure continuity of care across settings and among caregivers. Likewise,
failure to note that information and other key facts about the patient
in the medical record (i.e., diagnosis, treatment plan, known allergies,
etc.) may compromise the quality of anesthesia care and the safety of
the patient.

✒ *Compliance Tips*

Facilities must develop clear policies and standardized systems and protocols that require and encourage effective collaboration, communication, and information management. These policies must include a plan for patient care services that requires staff who steer patients through the continuum of care to

- assess patient needs upon admission;
- follow predetermined criteria for admission to all care settings (including, of course, those associated with anesthesia care);
- explain to patients and their families the costs of and alternatives to the planned course of treatment;
- ensure that discharges, transfers, and referrals do not disrupt treatment regimens;
- document in the medical record the caregiver's rationale for discharging, transferring, or referring a patient; and
- follow procedures to ensure that patient information is available to caregivers when they need it.

Facilities should constantly train and retrain caregivers to ensure that they are familiar with the policies and operate consistently and effectively within those systems. Whenever possible they should develop forms and checklists that reduce the chances that crucial patient information gets overlooked or miscommunicated. Humans make mistakes, and the more organizations can provide tools to support, prompt, and remind caregivers, the better off patients are likely to be. As with many other JCAHO standards, documentation of the steps taken to ensure compliance is a key part of demonstrating compliance. Organizations should be prepared to show surveyors written copies of their policies, procedures, and protocols. They should also take minutes and keep attendance lists at all training sessions so they can document their efforts and caregiver participation.

Anesthesia, sedation, and performance improvement

<table>
<tr><td align="center">RELEVANT STANDARDS

PI.3–PI.5

MS.8–MS.8.1.6

MS.8.3 & MS.8.4

IM.8

LD.1.4

LD.4.2–LD.4.3.2</td></tr>
</table>

New JCAHO standards outlining requirements for data-driven performance improvement took effect in 1999. They are designed to be less prescriptive than past requirements, emphasizing the importance of designing and maintaining a quality monitoring and improvement program that is tailored to the specific needs of an organization's patient population. They include fewer required performance measures and now identify suggested indicators that organizations can elect to monitor if there is a reason or need to do so. The remaining required measures target "high-risk, high-volume, problem-prone areas," including a number that relate to anesthesia and moderate or deep sedation:

- medication use;
- operative and other invasive and noninvasive procedures that can place patients at risk (e.g., CAT scans and MRIs);
- use of blood and blood products (*CAMH*, May 2000 update, PI.3.1.1).

Hospitals must assign, in writing, responsibility for implementing the improvement initiatives that result from PI analysis.

When relevant, performance-related information and findings must be forwarded to hospital leadership. The JCAHO expects hospital leaders to

- understand performance improvement (PI) techniques;
- adopt a specific approach to PI;
- require and encourage implementation of that approach as part of an effective PI program;
- allocate resources needed for effective PI; and
- participate in PI activities.

The JCAHO expects members of the medical staff to participate in PI analysis of all processes that are dependent upon licensed independent practitioners. The standards mention four specific processes, each of which relate to anesthesia or sedation:

- medical assessment and treatment of patients;
- use of medications;
- use of blood and blood components; and
- use of operative and other procedures (*CAMH*, August 2000 update, MS.8.1.4).

ORYX

Over the past three years, the JCAHO has been implementing what it calls the ORYX initiative, which is designed to

- allow the JCAHO to track hospital performance on an ongoing basis;
- encourage an ongoing, data-driven approach to performance improvement; and
- establish standardized "core measures" that allow the JCAHO to compare a hospital's performance against national norms.

The JCAHO has announced five core measures that hospitals began to track and report in 2000:

- acute myocardial infarction;
- congestive heart failure;
- pneumonia;
- pregnancy-related conditions; and
- surgical procedures and complications.

In addition, the JCAHO expects organizations to choose and report quarterly performance data for six additional measures that affect 30% of their patients.

Sentinel events

The current standards require organizations to analyze "undesirable patterns or trends in performance and sentinel events" (see Figure 2.7) and implement "changes that will lead to improved performance." The JCAHO identifies several types of incidents that organizations must analyze, including three that relate to anesthesia and sedation:

- significant adverse events associated with anesthesia care;
- significant adverse drug reactions; and
- significant medication errors (*CAMH*, August 1998 update, PI.4.3).

FIGURE
2.7

SENTINEL EVENTS

The JCAHO's sentinel events policy and standards targets unexpected incidents "involving death or serious physical or psychological injury, or the risk thereof" (*CAMH*, February 2000 update, APP-6). The JCAHO refers to such incidents as sentinel events and identifies five specific categories of event that warrant immediate action:

1. a patient suicide in a setting where the patient receives care around the clock
2. an infant abduction or discharge to the wrong family
3. a rape
4. a hemolytic reaction involving administration of blood or blood products having major blood group incompatibilities; or
5. surgery on the wrong patient or wrong body part

The stated goal of the policy and standards is to identify, investigate, and attempt to eliminate flaws in treatment systems and processes that put patients at risk. Any time patients die unexpectedly or experience a major, permanent loss of function that's not related to the natural course of their illnesses or conditions, organizations are encouraged to report the incident to the Joint Commission within five business days.[1] In addition, the JCAHO requires

---

[1] Reporting of sentinel events is currently voluntary. However, at the time this book was written, most experts advised organizations not to report sentinel events to the JCAHO for liability reasons. Because the Joint Commission does not have peer review status, it is possible that plaintiffs' attorneys could compel the JCAHO to reveal the information contained in verbal or written sentinel event reports. However, there is almost unanimous agreement that, whether they report them or not, it's important for healthcare organizations to respond to sentinel and other adverse events by investigating their root causes and redesigning systems and processes in an effort to prevent similar events from occurring.

continued

SENTINEL EVENTS

organizations to analyze such events no later than 45 days after learning of them.

Once that analysis is complete, organizations must take measurable steps designed to prevent similar incidents.

Organizations that do not complete sentinel event investigations within 45 days will be placed on accreditation watch, a designation that publicly indicates they experienced a sentinel event and have not cooperated with the JCAHO to reconcile it. If the organization does not complete an investigation within two weeks of going on accreditation watch, its accreditation will be revoked.

JCAHO surveyors are likely to ask for your definition of a sentinel event. They'll also want to discuss your methods for identifying and investigating them, and for designing systems improvements following those investigations. They are likely to ask organizations if they've experienced any sentinel events since their last survey and, since it's widely believed that all hospitals experience several per year, they'll react skeptically to organizations that claim they have not had any. Hospital leaders are responsible for ensuring that an organization establishes and implements systems for identifying and managing sentinel events.

✏️ *Compliance Tips*

Performance improvement must be a priority for all healthcare organizations, something they use proactively to fulfill their missions and to ensure the quality of care they provide. During interview sessions, surveyors will gauge how well physicians and hospital staff understand your organization's approach to PI (e.g., the FOCUS-PDCA method, the FADE method, etc.). They will want to see evidence that your PI program receives support and oversight at the highest levels. They will also want assurances that people at all levels of the organization and medical staff under-stand their PI roles and responsibilities and that they participate in improvement projects.

During interviews with caregivers, quality staff, leaders, and others, JCAHO surveyors may ask for examples of anesthesia-related incidents that your organization would consider adverse. They are also likely to ask about the performance indicators and monitoring mechanisms that your organization uses to identify such incidents (and related incidents, such as adverse drug reactions, medication errors, or unexpected admissions following outpatient surgery). They may also ask relevant personnel to discuss a recent anesthesia-related PI project undertaken within your organization. Make sure, therefore, that relevant members of the medical and hospital staffs are familiar with your policies and procedures for monitoring the quality of anesthesia care; moreover, formalize those and other PI policies and procedures by drafting a systemwide performance improvement plan. Your plan must address JCAHO requirements regarding monitoring and improvement of anesthesia care and other processes. In general, it should

- outline the performance indicators for sedation and anesthesia care (see Figure 2.8) and other clinical and nonclinical processes that your organization monitors;
- describe how your organization identifies and capitalizes on opportunities to improve sedation and anesthesia care and other clinical or nonclinical processes; and
- demonstrate your organization's commitment to PI as an ongoing, collaborative, and multidisciplinary process.

Effective PI programs are data-driven and produce measurable improvement initiatives, so JCAHO surveyors will also expect your plan to

- outline effective mechanisms for capturing information about quality of care (e.g., voluntary reporting by caregivers and/or regular auditing of medical records and performance-related databases);
- mandate the use of formal tools and techniques for evaluating performance data;
- require members of your PI taskforces to design and implement measurable improvement initiatives based on the data they have collected and analyzed; and
- require members of your PI taskforces to track the results of improvement initiatives and revise them, as needed.

FIGURE 2.8

ANESTHESIA INDICATORS

1. CNS complication within 2 postprocedure days

2. Peripheral neurologic deficit within 2 postprocedure days

3. Acute MI within 2 postprocedure days

4. Cardiac arrest within 2 postprocedure days

5. Respiratory arrest within 2 postprocedure days

6. Death within 2 postprocedure days

7. Unplanned admission within 1 postprocedure day of outpatient surgery

8. Unplanned admission to an ICU within 1 postprocedure day of surgery

9. Pulmonary edema within 1 post procedure day

10. Aspiration pneumonitis within 2 postprocedure days

11. Postural headache within 4 post procedure days of a spinal or epidural anesthetic

12. Dental injury during anesthetic care

13. Ocular injury during anesthetic care

Source: St. Joseph's Hospital and Medical Center, Phoenix, AZ.

An organization's PI plan is usually the primary source of documented evidence regarding compliance. However, other documents that will help to demonstrate compliance include an organization's mission or vision statement, minutes and attendance lists from PI task force meetings, and reports documenting the goals and results of improvement initiatives.

Anesthesia, sedation, and leadership

RELEVANT STANDARDS

LD.1.3.3 & LD.1.3.3.1

LD.1.6

LD.1.7 & LD.1.7.1

LD.2

LD.3

LD.3.2

LD.3.4

JCAHO leadership (LD) standards are relevant to this discussion of anesthesia and sedation because the Joint Commission expects hospital and medical staff leaders to

- decide which clinical services (including anesthesia and sedation) are consistent with the organization's and/or the medical executive committee's (MEC's) mission (see Figure 2.9) and should be available to patients;
- coordinate provision of those services within and across departments; and
- oversee and improve the quality of those services.

The JCAHO holds leaders responsible for ensuring that patients receive a comparable level of care in all treatment settings and from all practitioners within an organization. This requirement is particularly relevant to anesthesia because practitioners perform procedures involving anesthesia in a wide

FIGURE 2.9

SAMPLE MEC MISSION STATEMENT

The mission of the Executive Committee of the medical staff of
St. Joseph's Hospital and Medical Center is

- to provide proactive leadership for the organized medical
  staff in this rapidly changing healthcare environment.
- to ensure the provision of quality patient care and to
  measure the value of services rendered.
- to assure that physicians are appropriately credentialed
  for membership and privileged commensurate with their
  individual training and experience.
- to provide a forum to discuss and mediate other physician issues.
- to recommend action to the Board of Directors of Mercy
  Healthcare Arizona regarding items of concern to the
  medical staff.
- to assist in the strategic planning and direction taken by
  Mercy Healthcare Arizona and Catholic Healthcare West.

Source: St. Joseph's Hospital and Medical Center, Phoenix, AZ.

range of settings. It has become a more complicated leadership requirement
as the development of integrated health systems has expanded the range of
settings within organizations where patients receive anesthesia, sedation, and
other services.

As is the case in all clinical departments, the leadership of the anesthesia
department must prepare a written document outlining its goals and scope
of services. The JCAHO expects the department's goals to be consistent
with the organization's overall mission, and the scope of available anesthesia

services must adequately address the needs of the organization's patient population. Department leaders must provide support services and staffing that are consistent with the scope of services outlined.

 Compliance Tips

Organizations and anesthesia departments should be prepared to discuss their mission and scope of services with JCAHO surveyors. They must also develop policy and procedure documents that are consistent with the requirements outlined above, and they should document steps taken by hospital and medical staff leaders to ensure compliance with those policies and procedures.

In general, an organization's anesthesia policy should address the following leadership and management issues:

- the role of anesthesia services within the organization's overall goals, mission, and scope of services;
- credentialing and privileging requirements for anesthesia practitioners and others who administer moderate or deep sedation (see Chapter 3);
- systemwide protocols governing sedation and anesthesia care;
- guidelines for ensuring a comparable level of sedation and anesthesia care throughout the organization;
- expectations regarding collaboration between providers, departments, and specialties; and
- performance indicators and improvement requirements for sedation and anesthesia services.

Anesthesia, sedation, and the environment of care

RELEVANT STANDARDS

EC.1.3

EC.1.5–EC.1.9

EC.2.1

EC.2.2

EC.2.4–EC.2.9

EC.2.11–EC.2.14

While there is some unavoidable risk associated with anesthesia and sedation, facilities must take steps to minimize this risk. Patients receiving anesthesia or moderate or deep sedation may lose consciousness and be fully or partially immobilized. In those instances, they are dependent on medical equipment, skilled practitioners, and hospital staff to preserve their health and safety. When patients agree to undergo procedures involving sedation, for example, they trust that their caregivers will know how to react if they slip to a deeper level of sedation and that the equipment needed to keep them alive will be on hand and working reliably. Likewise, patients trust that facilities will have policies, procedures, and equipment in place to deal with fires, natural disasters, and other emergencies that have the potential to compromise their safety.

☞ *Compliance Tips*

To comply with the JCAHO's environment of care standards affecting anesthesia care, facilities must develop and implement management plans that outline key requirements (e.g., maintenance schedules, inspection schedules, testing/ drill schedules, staff training, etc.) in a number of areas, including

- safety;
- emergency preparedness (in case of fire, flood, tornado, riot, etc.);
- life safety;
- medical equipment (e.g., ventilators, etc.); and
- utility systems (e.g., electricity, water, telecommunications systems, etc.).

The requirements and policies outlined in these management plans must conform to state and federal laws, existing healthcare regulations, and current standards.

Organizations must hold training sessions and drills for all shifts to ensure that staff are prepared to respond to fires, equipment failures, power outages, and other emergencies that affect the environment of care and put patients at risk. They must document the occurrence and results of these tests, document staff participation in them, and address flaws in their management plan and/or deficiencies in staff knowledge or performance.

Managing human resources for anesthesia and sedation

```
RELEVANT STANDARDS
        HR.2
        HR.3
```

Facilities must be able to document that the practitioners and hospital staff involved in sedation and anesthesia care have enough training and experience to treat patients safely and effectively in all settings. Staffing in operating rooms, PACUs, and special-care units must be consistent with state and federal law, regulatory requirements, and a hospital's internal policies.

Hospital and physician leaders must develop systems to measure, maintain, and improve staff competency. Leaders involved directly in anesthesia care must assess staff competency in operating rooms, PACUs, and special-care units. They must plan and implement continuing medical education (CME) programs for the anesthesia department and should consider adopting the ASA's guidelines for CME (see pp. 142-144).

Staff training, competence, and experience must suit the needs of an organization's patient population, and caregiver competence must extend to all patients regardless of age or illness. In addition, all staff should be able to demonstrate that, for both high-risk, high-volume procedures and high-risk, low-volume procedures, they can competently treat patients of all ages served by a facility.

☛ *Compliance Tips*

Facilities should develop a policy on human resources that applies to all settings where and when providers administer sedation and anesthesia. The policy should require that

- members of the medical and hospital staff have sufficient training and experience to provide sedation and anesthesia services for the facility's patient population;

- the facility measures, maintains, and improves the performance of staff involved in sedation and anesthesia care; and
- the facility makes CME programs on sedation and anesthesia care available to all relevant staff.

The facility should also document actions and activities that indicate compliance with and enforcement of these policies.

Information management and anesthesia care

RELEVANT STANDARDS	
IM.5	IM.7.3.3
IM.7.3	IM.7.4
IM.7.3.1	IM.9

Because sedation and anesthesia are provided in different settings throughout the facility, medical records serve as the key source of information about a patient, and they are a key vehicle for ensuring the continuity and quality of care. Practitioners need information on past hospitalizations, surgeries, and procedures—especially as it pertains to a patient's past experiences with anesthesia or sedation. They also need to know about allergies, current diagnoses, results of relevant lab tests, and many other facts about a patient's condition or status—all of which affect decisions about anesthesia and sedation. Organizations must, in short, have policies and procedures in place for ensuring that the information in the medical record is

- accurate;
- up to date;

- formatted consistently so that caregivers can find what they need and are less likely to overlook key details; and
- available to practitioners and caregivers when they need it.

In ensuring caregiver access to patient information, however, organizations must also take documented steps to keep unauthorized individuals from accessing confidential information about patients.

Organizations must carefully monitor practitioner documentation to ensure that all pertinent information gets charted. For instance, practitioners must document all operative, diagnostic, and therapeutic procedures—including any use of anesthesia or sedation. Caregivers monitoring the patient's recovery from anesthesia or sedation must document the patient's vital signs and mental status. They also must document administration of medications, fluids, blood or blood products. And they are required to make note of unexpected events or complications, steps taken to resolve the situation, and the effect on the patient.

If a patient is discharged from the facility but requires continuing care, the patient's medical record must contain all information needed to guide that continuing care. Documents in the record should include summaries of diagnoses, procedures, medication use, allergies, and discharge instructions.

In addition to requiring organizations to manage patient information carefully, the JCAHO IM standards also insist that physicians and other caregivers have access to patient-care literature through medical journals, medical reference materials, and other such resources. These resources should include information that helps anesthesiologists, certified registered nurse anesthetists

(CRNAs), and other authorized caregivers provide safe, effective sedation and anesthesia care.

 Compliance Tips

To comply with the JCAHO IM standards affecting sedation and anesthesia care, organizations must develop and enforce policies and procedures that are consistent with the requirements outlined above. They should periodically audit medical records to ensure that the records include documentation for all necessary aspects of preanesthesia care, anesthesia care, and postanesthesia care. Organizations should also consider adopting the guidelines and standards laid out in the ASA's "Documentation of Anesthesia Care" (see pp. 145-146).

Infection control in anesthesia settings

RELEVANT STANDARDS

IC.2–IC.5

Due to the risks posed during anesthesia and sedation care by blood-borne infectious agents such as hepatitis and HIV and airborne infectious agents such as tuberculosis, healthcare facilities must vigilantly seek to prevent the transmission of disease from patient to patient or from patient to caregiver. A facility must dedicate educational resources to reducing the risks of transmission of infectious agents. It must also have policies for responding to and treating incidents that pose a significant threat of infection—like needle sticks and contact in other ways with potentially contaminated blood and other substances.

An organization's infection control policies must apply to all settings where sedation or anesthesia is administered. It should outline conditions of employment that are designed to reduce the risk of infection, such as mandatory tuberculosis screenings. Hospital and medical staff at risk of exposure to blood or bodily fluids should be encouraged to receive a hepatitis B vaccine, and personnel with active respiratory or cutaneous infections should not have direct contact with patients. The organization should also hold—and require employee participation in—periodic training sessions on infection control.

◗◆ *Compliance Tips*

Facilities must have written policies and procedures in place that address infection control and are consistent with guidelines developed by agencies such as the Centers for Disease Control and Prevention. Policies must conform with state and federal laws and regulations, and they should address the following issues:

- sterilization;
- disinfection;
- barrier precautions;
- handling sterile supplies;
- sanitation for rooms and supplies;
- hand washing;
- appropriate clothing, including eyewear and masks;
- handling and disposal of needles and other sharp objects; and
- adherence to standard infection control precautions.

Facilities must also document activities related to compliance with JCAHO IC standards, including enforcement actions and relevant training sessions.

Medical staff standards and anesthesia care

RELEVANT STANDARDS

MS.1–MS.1.1.3	MS.5.14–MS.5.15.7
MS.2.3	MS.6.2–MS.6.2.2.1
MS.2.3.2–MS.2.3.6	MS.6.4–MS.6.5.2
MS.2.5	MS.6.8–MS.7.2.1
MS.4–MS.4.2.1.15	

Anesthesiologists are members of a medical staff, the governing body for the licensed independent practitioners allowed to practice medicine in an organization. The JCAHO no longer requires organizations to have a single, organized medical staff, recognizing that managed care and the development of far-flung health systems makes that an unwieldy structure in many cases. However, the JCAHO still requires LIPs to practice within a governing structure, and it prohibits individual facilities from maintaining more than one medical staff.

The medical staff is responsible for the quality of services provided by its members and is accountable to an organization's board (or other governing body). Medical staff members must have delineated clinical privileges identifying the services and procedures they're authorized to order and perform (e.g., administration of anesthesia and/or sedation), and they are subject to the medical staff's bylaws, policies, rules, and regulations. Like all physician leaders, anesthesiologists must play an active role in medical staff leadership, quality monitoring, and performance improvement.

If an anesthesia department or group participates in graduate medical education programs, the organization's rules and regulations must outline requirements for medical staff supervision of interns, residents, and fellows. Medical staff members who serve as supervisors usually must countersign medical record entries written by house staff.

If certified registered nurse anesthetists (CRNAs) practice in an organization—whether they are self-employed or employed by the hospital or by other practitioners—they must practice in accordance with all laws and regulations, some of which vary by state. Some states, for instance, insist that an anesthesiologist supervise or direct all care that CRNAs provide. CRNAs must also comply with the internal policies and procedures of the facilities in which they practice, and when relevant, with the bylaws, rules, and regulations that govern the facility's medical staff. These medical staff governing documents should include criteria that allow for easy identification of instances when CRNAs must consult with a LIP. For instance, CRNAs may be allowed to perform all or part of a patient's history and physical—including the assessment of anesthesia risks—but medical staff policies and/or state and federal guidelines may require physician confirmation of the findings.

If a facility has an anesthesia department, it must have designated leadership—including a director with board certification or a comparable level of documented experience and skill. The chair or director of the anesthesia department—or of other departments that have need for anesthesia and sedation services (e.g., surgery, radiology, etc.)—is responsible for

- helping the facility identify the types of services needed to meet the patient population's needs;

- overseeing the clinical activities of the department;
- developing department policies and procedures,
- developing criteria for privileging;
- making recommendations regarding granting of clinical privileges; and
- ensuring the effectiveness of quality monitoring and performance improvement within the department.

Practitioners who are qualified to provide unsupervised patient care must have delineated clinical privileges that clearly describe the patient care services they are allowed to provide, and organizations must have systems in place to ensure that no practitioner orders or provides services and procedures that lie outside the scope of his or her privileges. Decisions to grant privileges should be based upon a review of specific criteria, including the specialty of the provider requesting privileges, the provider's training and experience, age-specific competencies, the risks associated with the procedures and services in question, and the requesting practitioner's ability to manage and address those risks.

Requirements regarding privileges extend to physicians and physician groups with exclusive contracts—a fact that is relevant to this discussion since anesthesiology is one of four service areas often provided on a contract basis (the other areas are radiology, pathology, and emergency medicine). The medical staff must define and approve a system for granting privileges to physicians who provide contracted services, and the medical staff's bylaws, credentials policy, and/or rules and regulations should explain this system.

For complicated or risky procedures, organizations should consider requiring evidence of specialized training and expertise. With regard to anesthesia and sedation, for instance, organizations might want to develop special criteria for practitioners seeking privileges to insert pulmonary artery catheters, provide anesthesia during open-heart surgery, perform invasive pain management procedures, or provide anesthesia care for infants.

In organizations that have clinical departments, LIPs must be assigned to departments that provide and monitor the services for which they have been granted privileges. If the organization does not have clinical departments, the medical staff's bylaws must outline formal processes for granting privileges and reviewing the quality of care provided by individual practitioners.

The JCAHO requires practitioners to participate in continuing medical education programs. Facilities must document their participation in these programs and must factor it into decisions regarding renewal of privileges and reappointment to the medical staff.

   Compliance Tips

Organizations must develop documents governing their medical staff (bylaws, policies and procedures, and rules and regulations) that are consistent with all requirements noted above. At bare minimum, the bylaws should

- outline the formal structure of the medical staff practicing within a facility or facilities;
- create a medical executive committee to oversee medical staff operations;
- outline a fair hearing and appeals process to protect the rights of medical staff members;
- address issues of unacceptable clinical practice, including disregard for rules, mental or physical impairment, disruptive behavior, and unethical behavior.

Beyond the bylaws, organizations should develop, implement, and enforce the following:

- a credentialing policy or manual;
- a clinical consultation policy;
- other relevant clinical policies;
- manuals outlining guidelines, policies, and methods for all clinical departments (including anesthesiology); and
- a plan for assessing physician performance and improvement.

All medical staff members must receive copies of these documents, as well as copies of significant revisions. The requirements and standards outlined in the documents governing medical staff must also be consistent with all relevant laws and regulations, and organizations must be able to document compliance with these documents. Indeed, staff failure to abide by organizational policies is one of the most common reasons that organizations receive Type I recommendations during JCAHO surveys.

The JCAHO standards do not require organizations to establish clinical departments. In fact, for small hospitals a nondepartmentalized approach can be quite effective. However, in facilities that do have clinical departments, department heads must be board certified or have an equivalent level of skill and experience. Organizations should be prepared to show JCAHO surveyors documented procedures for selecting department heads and a written job description outlining each department head's responsibility. They should also be able to demonstrate that they choose departmental leadership carefully.

Delineated clinical privileges must be individual-specific and based on demonstrated current competence; the JCAHO prohibits granting of blanket privileges to all physicians in a department or on a medical staff. Careful compliance with this requirement can help organizations begin to meet the JCAHO requirements calling for comparable levels of care.

Clinical privileges for contract physicians—a common status for anesthesiologists—are usually granted through normal or routine privileging channels. However, organizations should probably consult their legal counsel when determining what happens to those privileges if the contract is lost.

Finally, organizations must establish mechanisms to ensure that licensed independent practitioners order and perform only those services for which they have privileges, and that nonphysician practitioners (e.g., CRNAs) perform only those services outlined in their job descriptions or scope-of-service documents. To this end, organizations often circulate lists of practitioners who are authorized to order or perform risky or uncommon procedures; these lists and other mechanisms are commonly known as "point of patient" checks.

Pain management standards

RELEVANT STANDARDS	
RI.1.2	TX.5.4
RI.1.2.8	PF.1.7
PE.1.4	CC.6.1
TX.3.3	PI.3.1

With the realization that pain has long been undertreated in some institutions and with the recognition of pain as a major public health issue, new pain management standards became effective on January 1, 2001. It is important that anesthesia practitioners, because of their prominent role in pain management, have a clear understanding of these expectations.

Patients have a right to appropriate pain management. A facility's commitment to that right should be clearly enunciated to the patient, patient's family, facility staff, and physicians. The facility should ensure prompt recognition, evaluation, and treatment of pain by dedicated specialists using effective, modern techniques.

The facility's staff should be educated about adequate pain evaluation (including frequency, nature, duration, severity, and location of the pain) as well as its ongoing assessment during treatment. If present upon admission, pain should be evaluated at that time.

Age-specific techniques should be utilized for pain assessment; for example, a FACES (smile–frown) system for a pediatric service would be appropriate for children. Likewise, specialized methods of pain assessment may be necessary for patients with Alzheimer's disease.

Policies and procedures must support the safe and effective treatment of pain, as well as the proper storage, distribution, ordering, dispensing, and administration of controlled substances. Techniques such as patient-controlled analgesia (PCA) or epidural analgesia should be made available to appropriate candidates.

Following surgery, pain intensity and quality must be continuously assessed, treated, and then reassessed. Pain should play a role in the timing of a patient's discharge. Further, discharge planning should include provisions for follow-up treatment of symptoms such as pain.

Finally, the organization should collect data to monitor performance in pain assessment and treatment.

☞ *Compliance Tips*

To comply with the pain management standards, facilities should educate patients and their families (at the time of admission) that they have the right to appropriate pain management. With the assistance of anesthesia practitioners, some tertiary facilities will develop sophisticated multidisciplinary pain management teams offering advanced, comprehensive, noninvasive, and invasive techniques for pain management.

Hospital staff should participate in periodic education regarding pain recognition, assessment, and treatment—from the time of admission through the time of discharge and beyond. They should also be active participants in performance improvement initiatives to evaluate how well the organization cares for patients with pain.

Credentialing and Privileging Requirements

To help protect the safety of patients and ensure the quality of care they receive, hospitals and ambulatory care centers are required to assess and verify the credentials of the licensed independent practitioners (LIPs) who apply for appointment to that organization's medical staff. Credentialing involves verifying from primary sources that individual practitioners meet the organization's minimum requirements for appointment to the medical staff and have the medical education, training, and experience outlined on their applications. Appointment should last for no more than two years, at which point practitioners must apply for reappointment.

Once an organization verifies a practitioner's credentials and approves his or her application for membership on the medical staff, the organization must define the accepted scope of practice for that practitioner. This second process, known commonly as privileging, involves further review of experience and competence to determine whether the practitioner is qualified to perform the clinical procedures he or she has asked to perform (see Figure 3.1).

The permission to perform procedures and provide patient care services that an organization grants practitioners is known as delineated clinical privileges.

FIGURE 3.1	PRIVILEGING GUIDELINES FOR MODERATE ("CONSCIOUS") SEDATION	
Privilege Requested	**Minimum Formal Training**	**Required Previous Experience**
Moderate ("conscious") sedation	Successful completion of an accredited three-year residency in anesthesiology or Where appropriate, graduation from a nurse anesthesia educational program accredited by the American Association of Nurse Anesthetists' Council on Certification of Nurse Anesthesia Educational Programs (or the council's predecessor) or Successful completion of a residency (with or without a subspecialty fellowship) wherein the LIP received education, training, and experience to administer and/or supervise moderate sedation (this would apply to physicians other than anesthesiologists, such as pulmonologists, gastroenterologists, surgeons, or cardiologists)	Performance of moderate ("conscious") sedation for at least 50 patients over the past 12 months

Adapted from: Beverly E. Pybus, CMSC, The Privileging Quick Reference Guide, 2nd edition (Marblehead, MA: Opus Communications, 2001, pp. 41–43).

Before considering applications for a specific privilege, a healthcare facility's medical staff leadership and board must

- approve a plan for the facility to offer the procedure or service in question; and
- define criteria for determining which practitioners are qualified to perform the procedure or service in question.

Healthcare facilities must pay close attention to credentialing and privileging for anesthesia because it is a specialized, high-risk area of practice. The Joint Commission on Accreditation of Healthcare Organizations (JCAHO) recognizes these risks and has developed specific standards to govern anesthesia care in accredited facilities (see Chapter 2). The credentialing and privileging requirements included in these standards will receive additional attention in this chapter, along with a discussion on best practices for credentialing and privileging LIPs who provide sedation and anesthesia care.

Credentialing and privileging for sedation and anesthesia

The JCAHO requirements for credentialing and privileging apply, of course, to sedation and anesthesia care and the LIPs who provide it: anesthesiologists, surgeons, dentists, certified registered nurse anesthetists (CRNAs),[1] etc.

---

[1] Some credentialing experts say it is not always necessary to grant privileges to CRNAs because in many states and/or healthcare organizations, CRNAs are not considered LIPs, which makes them ineligible for medical staff membership. According to these experts, only LIPs—practitioners who by law and medical staff bylaws are allowed to direct and provide patient care without supervision—are required to secure appointment to a medical staff, and only medical staff members are required to have delineated clinical privileges. In states that do not recognize CRNAs as LIPs, or in organizations that make them hospital employees (like RNs) rather having them apply for appointment to the medical staff, it's not necessary to privilege CRNAs. Instead, the facility's human resources department should develop a CRNA job description and draft scope-of-practice documentation (outlining the specific patient-care services an individual CRNA can provide) for each CRNA authorized to practice in the facility.

They require that a facility's medical staff include only licensed physicians and/or appropriately licensed nonphysician practitioners who by law and the medical staff's bylaws are authorized to treat patients without supervision (state laws and/or organizational bylaws may not allow CRNAs to practice without supervision; see footnote 1). All medical staff members—including anesthesiologists—must have delineated privileges and are required to participate in performance improvement initiatives.

JCAHO standards for sedation and anesthesia care do not require the granting of privileges for the administration of minimal sedation (anxiolysis). Minimally sedated patients continue to respond normally to verbal commands, and they demonstrate normal cardiovascular and ventilatory function, although their cognitive function and coordination may be impaired. However, effective January 1, 2001, any deeper types of sedation—moderate ("conscious") sedation and deep sedation wherein ventilatory function may be impaired and spontaneous ventilation may be inadequate—require that such care be provided by qualified individuals (*CAMH*, August 2000 update, TX.2). In other words, practitioners wishing to provide such care must demonstrate appropriate credentials (including education, training, and experience) and privileges (as granted by the organization). Further, these practitioners must have the capability to "rescue" a patient whose level of sedation reaches a deeper stage. Although not a JCAHO requirement, certification in advanced cardiac life support (ACLS) may be part of institutional policies for credentialing and privileging for moderate sedation. Alternatively, courses in airway management techniques, including head, neck and mandible positioning, positive pressure mask ventilation, or endotracheal intubation may be specified for practitioners who are not anesthesia care providers. Further, practitioners utilizing deep sedation must be able to manage an unstable cardiovascular system (as well as manage patients who may not have adequate spontaneous ventilation). Again, ACLS certification or other courses or training in cardiopulmonary resuscitation or hemodynamic stabilization may be required. Performance improvement data demonstrating good patient care will help surveyors verify that your policies are effective.

The American Society of Anesthesiologists' "Guidelines for Delineation of Clinical Privileges in Anesthesiology" (see pp. 158-162) can serve as a valuable resource for organizations as they develop criteria upon which to judge requests for anesthesiology privileges. Many of those guidelines are consistent with the JCAHO requirements. Ultimately, however, organizations must evaluate requests for privileges by answering a series of key questions, including the following:

- Do our bylaws allow practitioners to perform the requested procedure(s)?
- Does the requesting practitioner have a current license to practice medicine?
- Do federal or state laws bar the practitioner from providing the requested service(s)?
- Is the practitioner's training or documented clinical experience consistent with his or her request for privileges?
- Does the practitioner's peer-review history and outcomes data indicate current competence?
- Is the practitioner mentally and physically able to provide the requested services?
- Do the practitioner's references and recommendations check out?

Is board certification required?

The JCAHO's medical staff standards require board certification or a comparable level of competence for department directors who were elected or appointed after January 1, 1992. In general, however, the JCAHO does not require anesthesiologists and other physicians seeking medical staff membership or delineated clinical privileges to be board certified. Nonetheless, many organizations view board certification as a strong indicator of skill and competence; they may choose to require board certification in the clinical specialty area(s) for which the privileges are granted—either for all practitioners applying or for less experienced practitioners (e.g., those who completed residencies after a certain date). Whether or not they choose to require board certification, organizations must apply their requirements uniformly to all practitioners.

Tailored privileges

Because some facilities provide anesthesia care that is complex or extensive, physicians at those facilities often must demonstrate competency in specialized areas. Included in these areas are

- high-risk or premature neonates;
- patients who are in critical condition or intensive care;
- patients experiencing acute or chronic pain;
- patients undergoing open-heart or transplant surgery;
- patients undergoing high-risk obstetrical procedures;
- patients undergoing other high-risk, specialized procedures for which practitioners need additional education, training, and experience.

In these circumstances, procedure-specific privileges are tailored to physicians with general privileges and the skills required for such highly specialized or technologically advanced care.

Credentialing for ambulatory centers

Credentialing and privileging requirements have been problematic for ambulatory centers; there, more and more procedures involving anesthesia and sedation are performed, and the range of settings and practitioners providing care may make it harder for organizations to ensure that patients receive a comparable level of care. The JCAHO can survey ambulatory facilities that are affiliated with hospitals under either its hospital or its ambulatory standards. In either case, the JCAHO standards for credentialing a practitioner are consistent:

- The center must have a defined process of credentialing, privileging, and appointment, with reappointment taking place at least every two years.
- Anesthesia practitioners must provide evidence of—and the facility must perform primary-source verification of—all relevant credentials, including licensure, education, training, and experience.

Free-standing centers have been known to accept at face value the verification activities of a hospital or to assume that membership on a hospital medical staff guarantees adequate credentials verification. Neither approach is acceptable. All organizations need to gather primary-source verification of practitioner credentials before granting appointments. They should do so with equal care and rigor, following four basic rules:

1. *Credential all practitioners.* The center's credentialing requirements and verification procedures must apply to all practitioners who apply for appointment to the medical staff and should be as stringent and thorough as a hospital's.
2. *Verify credentials through primary sources.* It is important that the facility get primary-source verification. Documents in the credential files can be copies, but the authenticity of those copies must have been verified by the organization holding the original.

3. *Use peer letters to verify credentials.* Many centers rely on peer letters—often from a hospital where a practitioner works—to check competency and conduct a quality review. That practice is acceptable, but those organizations should consider developing a form letter to help ensure that such surveys are consistent and comprehensive.

4. *Develop a quality review committee.* Anesthesiologists (and other practitioners with anesthesia and/or sedation privileges) should have relevant performance and outcomes data reviewed by a committee. The results of these reviews should affect decisions regarding appointment and reappointment.

Privileging in ambulatory centers

Because practitioners who provide sedation and/or anesthesia care (or other services) may perform different procedures in a hospital than in an ambulatory setting, their privileges must be facility-specific and reflect the care they will actually provide at the facility in question. Independent ambulatory centers must not carry over privileges granted by an unaffiliated hospital—or vice versa. Nor should a freestanding ambulatory center assume that because a practitioner was granted specific privileges by a hospital, he or she is competent to perform the same or similar procedures at the center. Practitioners must submit separate requests for privileges to each organization, and the organizations must evaluate each application separately and with equal care.

Furthermore, privileges should be practitioner-specific—especially for risky or advanced procedures. Since different practitioners have different levels of competence, organizations place patients at risk if they grant privileges simply because a practitioner has completed a specific residency training program. An anesthesiologist might be qualified to participate in many operative procedures, but not in open-heart surgery or in pediatric surgery. While it is becoming more acceptable to grant a specific set of "core privileges" to all practitioners in a clinical department, organizations must evaluate carefully the ability of practitioners to perform the procedures for which they request privileges.

Anesthesia care by nonphysician providers

There are approximately 24,000 certified registered nurse anesthetists in the United States. It is estimated that they participate in the delivery of 65% of the anesthetics administered to patients each year—most frequently as part of an anesthesia care team overseen by an anesthesiologist. To participate in the treatment of patients, CRNAs should have the following:

- certification by the AANA Council on Certification of Nurse Anesthetists;
- current state licensure as a registered nurse; and
- current professional liability insurance.

It is important that the work of CRNAs be consistent with state and federal mandates, as well as with the institution's bylaws and rules and regulations. At times, anesthesiologists will necessarily supervise or direct CRNAs; in some situations, other licensed independent practitioners—such as surgeons, dentists, or podiatrists—may supervise. If CRNAs are working without supervision or medical direction, it is important that state law and institutional policies allow them to do so. The JCAHO does not require that an anesthesiologist supervise CRNAs, only that

- the activity of CRNAs be consistent with state laws and the rules of the healthcare facility; and
- the quality of care provided by CRNAs, anesthesiologists, and any other authorized practitioners be comparable.

Developing policies on credentialing and privileging

To be effective, policies that address credentialing and privileging requirements for practitioners that provide anesthesia and sedation must take the following issues into account:

- state law;
- the medical needs of the facility's patient population; and
- the organization's mission and vision.

The policy must also address the minimum practitioner qualifications, scope of practice, and, if relevant, requirements regarding the supervision of nonphysician practitioners.

Performance improvement and peer review

The JCAHO requires the medical staff to be involved in performance improvement initiatives and to assume a leadership role in improving the level of care. Therefore, LIPs who administer anesthesia or sedation need to participate in relevant peer-review sessions, and they must work with performance improvement (PI) teams seeking to improve the quality of anesthesia care and related services.

Continuing medical education

Hospitals and ambulatory care centers generally do not require anesthesia practitioners to take part in more continuing medical education (CME) than is mandated by licensing bodies—although the JCAHO expects facilities to consider a practitioner's CME record during the reappointment process. Furthermore, healthcare facilities rarely develop internal CME programs and curricula. In choosing CME programs, therefore, anesthesia practitioners should ensure that the courses are approved by the American Medical Association—or, in the case of CRNAs, the American Nurses Association.

The JCAHO Survey

Editor's note: Although the basic agenda and structure of JCAHO surveys are usually quite uniform, each organization's survey experience tends to vary. Individual surveyors emphasize different issues, depending on their own areas of expertise and on the range of services offered by an organization or facility. This variability makes it a challenge to tell all organizations exactly what to expect during a JCAHO survey. Rather than do so here, the author has chosen to introduce organizations to key aspects of the survey process by briefly profiling one hospital's experience and observations.

Jan Magallanez, RN, entered the room as if she were coming home. And why not? Magallanez, then the coordinator for regulatory compliance for St. Joseph's Hospital and Medical Center in Phoenix, AZ had a *Comprehensive Accreditation Manual for Hospitals* under one arm and a stack of hospital policies and procedures under the other, and she was about to talk about JCAHO surveys. She was on familiar ground. A veteran of many JCAHO surveys, and one who has also logged many years of service in quality improvement, Magallanez is uniquely qualified to discuss the survey process—both generally and as it pertains to anesthesia-related standards.

"If you leave here understanding only one thing about JCAHO surveys and survey prep," she said as she bustled into the room, "let it be this: Know your policies and procedures; know your bylaws, your protocols, and your rules and regulations.

Study these documents carefully when you're preparing for a survey. JCAHO surveyors will, and they'll hold you to them."

Much of the advice that follows, whether it's in direct quotes or not, was gleaned from an in-depth discussion of the survey process with Magallanez.

The survey process

The JCAHO's survey team for hospitals usually includes a nurse, a physician, and an administrator—although this depends on the number of beds in a facility and the range of services it provides. The JCAHO may send more surveyors to very large facilities and fewer to very small facilities. Hospital surveys typically last three days but can take anywhere from two to five days; here again, the size of the facility is the key determining factor.

A person with a background in healthcare administration and a physician usually survey ambulatory facilities. Typical ambulatory surveys last two or three days, but they may take longer for organizations with multiple sites or facilities separated by long distances. Surveyors might not visit every site in an ambulatory network, but it is worth noting that, according to JCAHO documents, they always visit every site that offers anesthesia services.

How is anesthesia competence assessed?

JCAHO surveyors could address sedation- and anesthesia-related standards during many survey sessions (see Figure 4.1). Facilities, therefore, must be

FIGURE 4.1

SURVEY SESSIONS THAT ADDRESS SEDATION AND ANESTHESIA

Performance improvement overview

Document review

Leadership interview

Unit visits, including:

- anesthetizing locations

- ambulatory/outpatient clinics

- emergency services

- imaging services

- inpatient units (for hospitals)

- pharmacy services

Medical records review

Ethics interview

Medication use and nutrition care interview

Anesthesia, operative, and other invasive procedures interview

Infection control interview

Human resources interview

Medical staff credentials interview

Patient care interview

Medical staff leadership interview

Nursing leadership interview

Building tour

prepared to discuss sedation and anesthesia at just about any time. However, the document review, medical records review, unit visits, and building tour are likely to be the most crucial sessions. More than any others, these sessions allow surveyors to determine whether an organization's sedation- and anesthesia-related policies and procedures are consistent with all standards and regulations, and whether members of the medical and hospital staffs comply with the organization's policies and all other relevant requirements.

The opening conference

Surveys usually begin with an opening conference, which includes the survey team, the senior administrator from the facility being surveyed, and the facility staff person who is coordinating the survey agenda and activities. This conference gives all parties an opportunity to review and, if necessary, discuss revisions to the survey agenda.

The PI overview

After the opening conference, JCAHO surveyors usually begin the performance improvement overview. During this session, they will want to see evidence that your facility has a systematic, multidisciplinary program for improving performance. This is a crucial session and should include key members of senior management and physician leaders who participate in performance improvement activities. Furthermore, an organization's performance improvement plan and program should address issues related to anesthesia and sedation, since these services are risky and can have a significant impact on outcomes and quality of care. Participants at the PI overview should be ready to discuss data-driven initiatives designed to improve the quality of sedation and anesthesia care— including responses to sentinel events (see p. 55) that involved anesthesia or sedation.

Document and records reviews

As with the PI overview, surveyors generally hold the document review session on the first day of a survey. "The survey team will want to see your bylaws, policies and procedures, and any other functional documents your facility may have," said Magallanez. "For example, they may want to see your informed consent policy. Then they will want to see how you comply with the policy." Policies that are important in the context of anesthesia and sedation include those regarding

- informed consent;
- preanesthesia assessments;
- delineation of clinical privileges;
- provision of comparable levels of care; and
- medication use and control—especially for controlled substances.

Surveyors will review key documents during this session—such as the preanesthesia and postanesthesia assessment records, anesthesia records, and consent agreements. It often makes sense for hospitals to audit these documents in advance of a survey to identify deficiencies and improve their documentation processes as needed. "Several years ago, our hospital became concerned that some preoperative assessments lacked the actual patient weights and baseline oxygen-saturation data," Magallanez said, explaining how audits help St. Joseph's prepare for surveys. "By performing a medical records review, and through a subsequent change in the preoperative nursing assessment process, we were able to improve documentation dramatically."

"The chart review also revealed that some of our anesthesia preoperative assessments did not include a physical status classification or list medication allergies," she added. "Working through the anesthesia committee, we modified the anesthesia record and distributed educational information to the staff anesthesiologists, which helped to dramatically raise our compliance with this JCAHO expectation. We also gained an additional benefit from this process through improved documentation on informed consent for anesthesia."

During the medical records review, surveyors search for evidence that staff consistently document the following:

- preoperative history and physical;
- diagnosis;
- preanesthesia assessment;
- anesthesia or sedation plan;
- a determination by an LIP that the anesthesia or sedation is appropriate for the patient;
- a nursing care plan;
- patient reevaluation prior to the anesthesia or sedation;
- patient monitoring during the anesthesia or sedation;
- postanesthesia monitoring; and
- patient discharge from the postanesthesia care unit by an LIP or in accordance with uniform medical staff criteria.

Unit visits

To get a first-hand look at patient care procedures, surveyors will visit wards and units to observe and speak with patients, physicians, and hospital staff. They will want to see whether staff consistently follow policies and procedures. They'll note whether staff effectively educate patients and families about sedation and anesthesia and about alternative treatment options. They'll be particularly interested to know whether staff take special educational needs into account, such as language or cultural differences. They'll also check to see whether qualified practitioners assess patients, formulate sedation or anesthesia plans, and obtain consent.

In the document and record review sessions, the JCAHO wants to see that a facility has clear guidelines for patient care during sedation or anesthesia. During unit visits, surveyors determine how well staff understand and follow these guidelines, the idea being that diligent compliance with effective policies usually translates into safe, effective anesthesia care. "When the Harvard Medical School developed its 'Standards for Intraoperative Monitoring,'" said Magallanez, "our anesthesia department quickly incorporated them into its departmental rules and guidelines. Not only did this help us comply with the JCAHO standards, our physicians and staff are convinced it resulted in better patient care."

EC interview and building tours

During interviews with staff responsible for the environment of care (EC) and during building tours, JCAHO surveyors will check whether a facility has and follows a preventive maintenance schedule for anesthesia equipment. They will review the preventive maintenance logs, which document that medical equipment and devices are tested and inspected appropriately. They will also need to see evidence that, when a problem or malfunction exists, the situation is documented and corrected.

"During one survey," Magallanez noted, "our chairman of anesthesia was impressed that the physician surveyor focused primarily on preventive maintenance for anesthesia equipment. The surveyor wanted to see documentation for two years' worth of service and maintenance for each of the 30 machines. Fortunately, we had it, and our the records were complete, accurate, and in compliance with the JCAHO standards and manufacturer recommendations."

Surveyors will also focus on other areas of facility management. For example:

- The facility must ensure that anesthesia-care sites have adequate supplies of oxygen, and it must identify the people responsible for maintaining that supply;
- The facility must show that it handles and disposes of contaminated waste and sharp objects appropriately;
- Staff must demonstrate that they know how to respond to emergencies (fires, natural disasters, etc.) that might require them to implement evacuation plans or perform other duties and procedures that aren't part of their normal work day; and
- The facility must be able to show that it is prepared for power failures and that it maintains back-up equipment in ways that minimize the risk to patients during an outage.

Checking for comparable levels of care

"The survey team will visit settings in the hospital where sedation or anesthesia is administered," said Magallanez. "The team will want to see how a facility meets the requirement mandating comparable levels of care." To do so, surveyors will

- visit your preoperative or preprocedure holding area and ask to review procedures and documentation for history and physical examinations, preanesthesia assessments, and anesthesia plans—all of which must be completed before the patient enters the operative suite;

- look for comparable monitoring equipment, staffing, and resuscitative equipment in various settings;
- check to ensure that uniform policies govern anesthesia care and medication use across all settings; and
- look for evidence that only practitioners with appropriate privileges and training order and/or administer anesthesia or moderate or deep sedation.

The survey team also reviews policies governing maintenance of patient-monitoring and anesthesia-delivery systems for evidence that facilities provide a comparable level of care. "Years ago, when capnometry became available in our inpatient operating rooms, this monitoring technology was not immediately in use in our outpatient surgery center," said Magallanez. "While preparing for a survey, we realized this meant we were not meeting the standard for comparable levels of care, so we took steps to provide a capnometer for each ambulatory operating room—and in x-ray rooms, the cardiac catheterization laboratory, and the MRI unit."

Magallanez also noted that providing a comparable level of care also became an issue when the hospital opened a lithotripsy unit several years ago. Patients were given anesthesia in the unit, then taken to a recovery area. However, they were not being discharged according to the same criteria used in the operating room's postanesthesia care unit (PACU). With the assistance of the head nurse from the surgical PACU, the hospital implemented uniform discharge criteria for the lithotripsy unit and operating rooms, thereby eliminating a source of variation in the provision of post-anesthesia care.

Hospital develops uniform sedation policy

Editor's note: Several years ago, with a JCAHO survey approaching, officials at St. Joseph's Hospital and Medical Center in Phoenix, AZ, realized that their facility was probably not in compliance with the JCAHO's comparable care requirements because it did not have a single policy governing sedation across the facility. In preparation for that survey, they launched an initiative to shape such a policy. The author has profiled their efforts here, to illustrate some of the benefits of effective survey preparation.

St. Joseph's Hospital and Medical Center in Phoenix, AZ, is an urban, tertiary healthcare facility with more than 550 licensed acute beds and an active medical staff of 559 physicians. The hospital provides diagnostic or therapeutic procedures requiring sedation or anesthesia at a wide variety of locations within the facility, including

- the eye and dental clinics;
- the MRI, CT, and radiology suites;
- the endoscopy and lithotripsy units;
- the radiation therapy department;
- the emergency room;
- the cardiac catheterization lab; and
- the ambulatory and inpatient operating departments.

Before 1994, each location listed above had a separate sedation policy. Each unit credentialed its own practitioners, developed dosage guidelines, provided oversight within its clinical areas, developed patient-monitoring and staffing guidelines, and implemented its own quality assurance and quality improvement programs.

The challenge

These location-specific policies and programs became a problem when the JCAHO developed anesthesia standards that mandate a comparable level of care throughout an organization. The hospital decided to use performance improvement (PI) tools and techniques to develop a single policy that would help them meet that comparable-care requirement.

The process

The president of the medical staff and the chairman of the medical staff's quality assurance committee created a task force to develop the uniform policy and designated an anesthesiologist to chair it. Other physician members on the task force included a radiologist, a dentist, a surgeon, a pediatrician, a pediatric intensivist, a pulmonologist, a gastroenterologist, and a cardiologist. The vice president of nursing, the quality improvement coordinators for ambulatory services and case management, and the chief clinical pharmacist also served on the task force.

The task force gathered the sedation policies and dosage guidelines that existed in the facility and analyzed existing utilization and performance data for sedation. It reviewed current literature concerning sedation, including the latest usage and dosage information for sedation-related medications. The task force took into account the role of sedation in all relevant clinical specialty areas and sought input from interested medical staff members in those areas.

The task force developed a drug dosage guideline table that included drugs and dosages for sedation. It also developed procedures to follow when sedation was given within these guidelines and outlined requirements regarding

- credentialing and privileging;
- staffing requirements;
- ongoing educational requirements (ACLS certification) of practitioners and staff;
- responsibilities of practitioners and staff;
- preanesthesia/presedation assessment;
- monitoring immediately before, during, and following the sedation;
- equipment available for monitoring, care, and resuscitation;
- postanesthetic/postsedation care and monitoring;
- unit or facility discharge by uniform criteria approved by the medical staff.

The guidelines were to be applied uniformly throughout the facility, regardless of setting or practitioner involved. They also required practitioners to notify the performance improvement department of any adverse events or trends. This requirement allowed the PI staff to track performance and identify needs and opportunities for improvement.

Relevant clinical departments and committees reviewed the new guidelines. Then, the medical executive committee and the hospital board reviewed the policy and gave final approval, opening the way for facility-wide implementation.

The outcome

St. Joseph's new policy ensured comparable levels of care for patients receiving sedation and anesthesia. It also established a mechanism for identifying performance trends, adverse events, and improvement opportunities. It is worth noting that the hospital took a multidisciplinary, interdepartmental approach to developing its policy and procedures, which included the following key steps:

- The *ad hoc* task force incorporated suggestions and input from all clinical disciplines that rely on anesthesia or sedation;
- Relevant clinical committees reviewed the draft policy and helped create the final document; and
- The clinical committees, the medical executive committee, and the hospital board reviewed and approved the new policy.

The inclusive approach went a long way toward ensuring the effectiveness of the policy and procedures implemented, because it ensured that all relevant viewpoints helped shape it. It also helped St. Joseph's comply with key JCAHO requirements regarding multidisciplinary involvement in performance improvement initiatives.

Performance Monitoring and Improvement

This chapter outlines data-driven strategies for monitoring and improving the performance of practitioners involved in anesthesia care. It outlines basic quality improvement tools and techniques and discusses how a practical quality-tracking report can help anesthesia departments build effective quality monitoring and improvement programs.

What is quality?

The term *quality* means different things to different people. To some, it implies adherence to a predetermined set of production standards. To others, it means the maintenance of a high level of service and customer satisfaction. Whatever your definition, monitoring and improving quality are crucial functions within healthcare organizations and should be continuous activities in the anesthesia department, as well as any other clinical or nonclinical department whose operations affect patient care and patient safety.

What is continuous quality improvement?

Continuous quality improvement (CQI) is a data-driven process for improving performance and is fueled by an open-minded, thoughtful evaluation of opportunities for change. It involves looking proactively at an organization's functions, services, and products and asking, "How can we do better?" At its most basic level, CQI is a tool for responding to existing problems, but the ideal quality-management system uses CQI techniques to prevent problems or to uncover opportunities for improving an otherwise acceptable status quo.

The terms *continuous quality improvement* and *quality assurance* (QA) are often used interchangeably, but they are different concepts. QA involves looking for problems retrospectively. It often assumes that some amount of error or imperfection is inevitable and, therefore, acceptable. Embracing CQI means welcoming an atmosphere that not only encourages change but actively seeks it out. It means accepting the notion that processes and products can always be improved through analysis, and that each error, defect, complaint, or inefficiency— no matter how small—represents an opportunity for improvement.

Choosing quality indicators

Once a healthcare facility or an anesthesia department defines its CQI goals and expectations, it must establish reliable methods for measuring its actual performance against those goals. That means identifying quality indicators and performance criteria that are relevant to core performance expectations— your own expectations and those of patients and other "customer" groups.

Focus on "customers"
Identifying the expectations of "customers" is crucial to the selection of indicators; if you don't know what they want or need, you may monitor the wrong things and make ineffective improvement decisions. For instance, in addition

to monitoring outcomes and patient safety, an anesthesia department's CQI team might choose to monitor patient satisfaction. As part of an effort to do so, team members might track the number of patients who receive drugs to treat nausea in the postanesthesia care unit (PACU)—working under the assumption that nausea leads to dissatisfaction and that effective use of drugs to treat nausea will translate into improved satisfaction. However, if patients expect to experience some nausea following an operative procedure, they may not react to it in an overly negative way. Rather than tracking usage of antinausea medications, therefore, a more meaningful indicator might be the number of patients who complain about nausea. Once the frequency of complaints crosses a predetermined threshold, the CQI team might look at secondary data sets—such usage rates for drugs that treat nausea—to generate strategies for addressing the problem. But in this instance, drug usage might not be an effective primary indicator.

Identifying improvement opportunities

Once indicators have been chosen, CQI teams need to create a mechanism for organizing indicator data in meaningful ways. Fortunately, there's no need to recreate the wheel. Finance departments in many healthcare facilities use a brief report (see Figure 5.1) to monitor the financial performance of the facility. This report organizes data in a way that allows the facility to

- compare current performance against past performance; and/or
- determine whether current performance is in line with the organization's budgeted goals and expectations.

This reporting format is particularly effective because it allows analysts to draw conclusions quickly about basic performance (to perform a "pulse check," so to speak) while also facilitating more in-depth analysis and the formation of more sophisticated conclusions regarding performance.

FIGURE
5.1

FINANCIAL PERFORMANCE REPORT

Indicators	January	February	Current month	Same month last year	Budget
Avg daily census	75	74	76	76	75
Total patient days	7,000	6,800	7,100	7,300	7,000
Average length of stay	6.2	6.1	6.0	6.4	6.2
E.R. visits	1,600	1,700	1,600	1,550	1,550
Cash on hand ($)	175,000	165,000	170,000	163,000	172,000
Age of A/R (days)	56	53	53	62	55
Interest on investments (%)	10.0	9.0	9.2	15.5	10.0
Write-offs ($)	7,000	6,800	7,100	7,300	7,000
Accts receivable ($)	155,650	150,000	152,000	153,000	150,000
Accts payable ($)	75,650	79,000	62,000	78,000	65,000
Incorrect bills	18	18	16	15	N/A
Lost charges ($)	1,700	1,800	1,700	1,600	N/A

Understanding the financial model

The report does not attempt to address every deficiency or problem that surfaces in a busy finance department; for instance, the steps taken to address a few incorrect bills might not appear in the report because the deficiency rate is not significant enough. Instead, the report tracks bigger-picture performance indicators—those that will demonstrate whether the facility's overall financial performance is on target. If the report suggests that the facility's financial performance is lagging, it would trigger more detailed analysis aimed at identifying potential causes and corrective actions.

Applying the financial model to anesthesia and sedation

Anesthesia departments can use this same reporting format to track performance indicators that are relevant to the provision of anesthesia and sedation—and, more importantly, to shape improvement initiatives when quality lags (see Figure 5.2). The first step, of course, involves the development of appropriate indicators that monitor the volume or frequency of key performance-related events or that reflect perceptions regarding quality and performance.

Volume indicators simply identify how often something happens. In the context of anesthesia care, such indicators might track basic procedures—for example, the total number of

- central venous line placements;
- intraoperative blood transfusions; or
- epidural anesthetics for cesarean deliveries.

Volume indicators might also track events that are indicative of adverse events, such as

FIGURE 5.2

PERFORMANCE REPORT: ANESTHESIA & SEDATION

Anesthesia & Sedation

Indicators / Occurrences	Jan	Feb	Mar	Apr	May	June	July	Aug	Sept	Oct	Nov	Dec	Dept. Standard
General anesthesia													
Regional anesthesia													
Monitored anesthesia care													
Sedation cases													
Sedation cases with loss of independent ventilatory function													
Codes responded to													
Catheter placements													
Pain mgmt. procedures													
Adverse event reports													
Patient complaints													
Practitioner complaints													
Related infections													
Late assessments													
PACU discharges by LIP													
Late H&Ps													
Related mortalities													
Poorly documented transfusions													

FIGURE 5.2 *continued*

PERFORMANCE REPORT: ANESTHESIA & SEDATION

Indicators / Occurrences	Jan	Feb	Mar	Apr	May	June	July	Aug	Sept	Oct	Nov	Dec	Dept. Standard
Perioperative myocardial infarctions													
Postdural headaches													
Patients with damaged teeth													
Patients with post-op neurological effects													
Patients with post-op pneumonia													
Patients with post-op aspiration													
Relevant malpractice claims													
Relevant delayed recoveries													
Relevant delays in surgery													
Procedure delays													
Procedure cancellation													

- unexpected hospital admissions following outpatient surgery;
- instances calling for reintubation of a patient in the PACU; or
- pneumothoraces associated with placement of central venous pressure catheters.

This second category of volume indicators correlates directly with performance quality, which makes such indicators particularly useful. However, it is also important for organizations to monitor perceptions regarding quality. This generally involves identification of indicators that gauge patient and employee satisfaction and development of vehicles (e.g., surveys, suggestion boxes, etc.) that can capture relevant data and highlight improvement opportunities.

Implementing improvement initiatives

Healthcare organizations and individual clinical departments should not treat operational changes lightly—particularly when they affect quality of care. Once improvement opportunities surface, CQI teams need to think carefully about how to act on them, and they must monitor the results of their improvement initiatives—to ensure both that they're having the effects intended and that they're not having an unexpected impact elsewhere along the continuum of care. Whenever possible, organizations may want to stage small-scale trials to test change initiatives before enacting them generally. What follows is a discussion of a structured approach to CQI that makes use of such trials.

The FOCUS PDCA approach

The FOCUS PDCA approach to quality improvement builds upon one of the earliest systematic techniques for controlling quality: the PDCA method (see

Figure 5.3). Walter Shewart, a quality pioneer in manufacturing circles, developed the PDCA method in the 1920s. During the 1950s, W. Edwards Deming popularized the approach among Japanese manufacturers—which is why it is sometimes called "The Deming Cycle."

Organizations can apply Shewart's and Deming's four-stage PDCA process

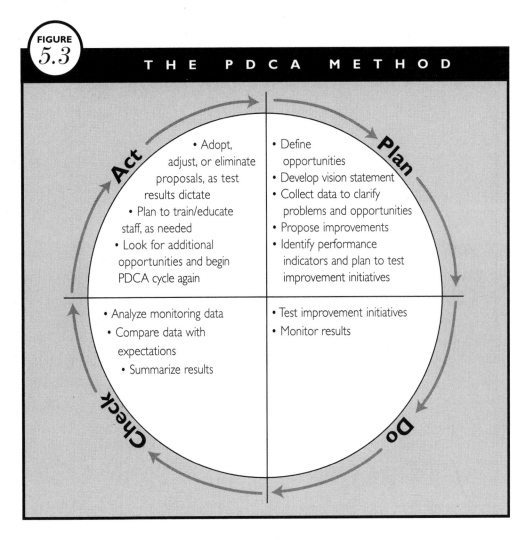

FIGURE 5.3

THE PDCA METHOD

Act
- Adopt, adjust, or eliminate proposals, as test results dictate
- Plan to train/educate staff, as needed
- Look for additional opportunities and begin PDCA cycle again

Plan
- Define opportunities
- Develop vision statement
- Collect data to clarify problems and opportunities
- Propose improvements
- Identify performance indicators and plan to test improvement initiatives

Check
- Analyze monitoring data
- Compare data with expectations
- Summarize results

Do
- Test improvement initiatives
- Monitor results

proactively, but most view it as a reactive tool. Rather than using the process to assess and improve systems before a problem arises, they generally wait for signs of an adverse event or outcome and apply the PDCA method in response.

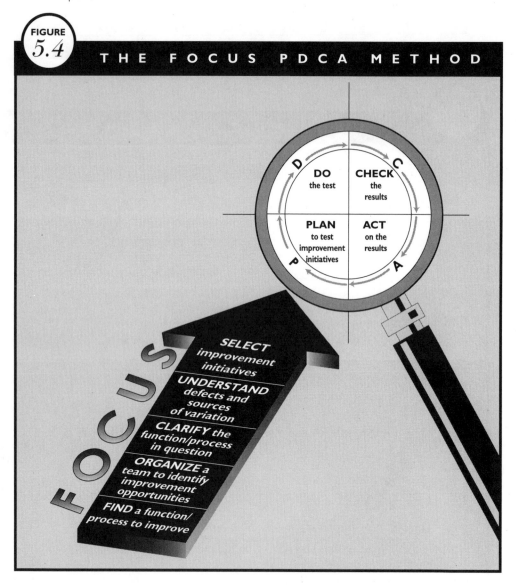

FIGURE 5.4

THE FOCUS PDCA METHOD

DO the test

CHECK the results

PLAN to test improvement initiatives

ACT on the results

FOCUS

SELECT improvement initiatives

UNDERSTAND defects and sources of variation

CLARIFY the function/process in question

ORGANIZE a team to identify improvement opportunities

FIND a function/process to improve

FOCUS PDCA (see Figure 5.4) makes the proactive potential of the basic Shewart/Deming approach more explicit. In the process, it turns an effective quality-assurance tool into a powerful vehicle for continuous quality improvement. FOCUS PDCA is founded upon the assumption that a system can always run better; it challenges organizations to seek out improvement opportunities.

FOCUS: Find a process to improve

Ideally, healthcare organizations seek to establish mechanisms that reveal systemic defects or performance variations before quality suffers dramatically— mechanisms such as performance measures, monitoring systems, and an organizational culture that seeks out opportunities to change and improve. This kind of speculative analysis of anesthesia-care processes is well suited to helping department leaders and performance-monitoring teams correct systemic flaws before a serious incident puts patients, practitioners' careers, or an organization's reputation at risk.

FOCUS: Organize a team

Whether analysis teams are responsible for reactive investigation of a quality lapse or proactive identification of improvement opportunities, team members must have firsthand knowledge of the processes they are evaluating. Physicians with anesthesiology privileges, pharmacists, CRNAs, and registered nurses (especially RNs who administer sedatives and/or care for patients who receive anesthesia or sedation) should serve on CQI teams that address performance issues related to anesthesia and sedation. It also helps to involve administrative staff who understand CQI, statistical analysis, and/or the standards and regulations governing anesthesia and sedation. Finally, it is important for CQI teams to have decision-making authority and the ability to implement change, which makes the support of physician and hospital leaders crucial.

FOCUS: Clarify the process in question

Once an organization has identified key processes and organized a team to improve them, that team must carefully chart each step in the processes under examination. Recruiting team members who have a relevant mix of skills and expertise is an important first step. Flow charts that diagram the processes under examination can assist in the clarification process—as can interviews with, and surveys of, others involved in the processes.

FOCUS: Understand sources of variation

Clarifying each step in the process under investigation often helps the team begin to identify gaps, inefficiencies, defects, and risk areas—aspects of that process that seem likely to prompt performance variations. As they identify such flaws, team members need to ask themselves what, if anything, caused them. They must peel away as many causal layers as possible to uncover the root causes of performance variation.

FOCUS: Select improvement initiatives

Once teams understand the root causes of performance variation, they can begin to propose and design improvement initiatives. If teams develop a number of improvement proposals, or if they locate more systemic defects than they can realistically address, they need to prioritize. Team members should implement the improvement proposals that seem most promising or likely to have the most far-reaching effects.

PDCA: Data-driven change, measurable improvement

Healthcare organizations often approach change cautiously—and they should. Not all change leads to improvement, as Coca Cola learned when it released New Coke. But, unlike miscalculations in the business sector, misguided change in healthcare can place patients' lives in jeopardy. That's why it is crucial for healthcare organizations to monitor the results of improvement initiatives. If an initiative is not having the expected effect, or if it is having unexpected impact on other functions, organizations need to react quickly before the quality of patient care suffers significantly. The FOCUS phase of FOCUS PDCA provides a systematic, data-driven method for identifying improvement opportunities and designing change initiatives. The PDCA phase, described below, offers a proven method for implementing, evaluating, and adjusting initiatives, as needed, to make them as effective as possible.

PDCA: Plan to test/implement initiatives

Organizations often hold small-scale trials of a new process before implementing it widely. Sometimes called pilots, these test runs allow the organization to control or minimize the impact of a new method or procedure until there is clear evidence that the effects will be positive. Also, because they are limited in scope, trial runs often are more cost-effective than immediate, full-scale implementation of new policies and procedures.

Regardless of whether improvement teams choose to stage a trial, it is crucial that its members develop an action plan to guide their implementation and evaluation efforts (see Figure 5.5, p. 118). Effective action plans include seven basic components:

1. a mission statement that defines a specific, measurable objective;
2. an overview of tactics (change initiatives) that will help the team fulfill its objective;
3. clear, measurable expectations regarding results;
4. identification of performance indicators to measure results against expectations;

FIGURE 5.5

SAMPLE CQI ACTION PLAN

CQI Action Plan

Facilitator: **Launch Date:**

Mission Statement:

Improvement Tactics	Performance Indicators	Data Sources & Collection Methods	Analysis Due	Results & Recommendations
tactic: coordinator: targeted result:			prelim: final:	
tactic: coordinator: targeted result:			prelim: final:	
tactic: coordinator: targeted result:			prelim: final:	
tactic: coordinator: targeted result:			prelim: final:	

5. an explanation of data-collection mechanisms to be used in monitoring those indicators;

6. designations of responsibility for each action item or tactic in the plan; and

7. a timeline for staging preliminary and final assessments of each change initiative.

The planning process should include consideration of possible direct and indirect effects of a change initiative. Patient-care functions and processes are often interconnected, but not always in obvious ways. Adjustments to one function may produce effects in others. If team members don't commit time and resources to anticipating, addressing, and monitoring such unexpected or less obvious effects, the negative results in one area could neutralize important gains in another.

PDCA: Do the test/implement change

Once the team has outlined its tactics, assigned responsibilities, and settled on a timeline for each initiative, it is ready to implement the proposed changes. Depending on the size of the team and the number of initiatives under consideration, team members may want to separate themselves into smaller work groups for this phase. If they do so, periodic meetings of the full team will help keep the overall project on track, allow work group members to seek input from others, and provide a forum for reporting and discussing preliminary findings.

PDCA: Check the results

When the trial run (or the initial phase of a full-scale implementation) is complete, the team should analyze the performance monitoring data that it collected and compare its findings against its improvement goals. Change initiatives should never go unmonitored or unanalyzed.

Chapter Five

PDCA: Act on the results

If the results of an improvement plan are unsatisfactory, the team may need to reconsider or refine proposed changes and repeat the PDCA cycle. If, however, change initiatives meet or exceed expectations, team members should take steps to enact them across the organization. Enactment may involve working with hospital and medical staff leaders to revise existing policies and procedures, developing staff-retraining initiatives, and other activities.

Sample Sedation Policy and Consent Forms

The sample moderate ("conscious") sedation policy as well as sample consent forms for anesthesia, blood or blood administration, and operative or invasive procedures have been provided courtesy of The Greeley Company in Marblehead, MA. Organizations are encouraged to use these documents as a model when developing or evaluating their own policies and forms governing moderate sedation and anesthesia.

Moderate ("Conscious") Sedation Policy

1. Policy

Moderate sedation, also known as conscious sedation or analgesia, is produced by the administration of drugs to dull or reduce a patient's pain and awareness during diagnostic or therapeutic procedures. The dose of the drug or drugs given is not intended to cause the patient to lose the ability to independently and continuously maintain a patent airway or respond appropriately to physical stimulation. However, since sedation is a continuum, this policy is designed to provide a safe level of care to patients who slip into a deeper level of sedation and lose their ability to maintain independent ventilatory function.

2. Definitions[1]

Minimal sedation (anxiolysis): A drug-induced state during which patients respond normally to verbal commands. Although cognitive function and coordination may be impaired, ventilatory and cardiovascular functions are unaffected. Medication used for this purpose and for sedation of mechanically ventilated patients or for urgent/emergent endotracheal intubation is covered by separate protocols.

Moderate sedation/analgesia ("conscious" sedation): A drug-induced depression of consciousness during which patients respond purposefully to verbal commands, either alone or accompanied by light tactile stimulation. No interventions are required to maintain a patent airway, and spontaneous ventilation is adequate. Cardiovascular function is usually maintained.

---

[1] Note: The definitions in this policy are based on Continuum of Depth of Sedation Definition of General Anesthesia and Levels of Sedation/Analgesia ©2001 of the American Society of Anesthesiologists (see pp. 140-141).

Deep sedation/analgesia: A drug-induced depression of consciousness during which patients cannot be easily aroused but respond purposefully following repeated or painful stimulation. The ability to independently maintain ventilatory function maybe impaired. Patients may require assistance in maintaining a patent airway and spontaneous ventilation may be inadequate. Cardiovascular function is usually maintained. Deep sedation and anesthesia is restricted to use by an anesthesia provider.

Anesthesia: Consists of general anesthesia and spinal or major regional anesthesia. It does not include local anesthesia. General anesthesia is a drug-induced loss of consciousness during which patients are not arousable, even by painful stimulation. The ability to independently maintain ventilatory function is often impaired. Patients often require assistance in maintaining a patent airway, and positive pressure ventilation may be required because of depressed spontaneous ventilation or drug-induced depression of neuromuscular function. Cardiovascular function may be impaired.

Privileging criteria and qualifications

Only a qualified physician—one who is trained in professional standards and techniques to administer pharmacologic agents to predictably achieve desired levels of sedation and to monitor patients carefully in order to maintain them at the desired level of sedation, and who meets the criteria set by the medical executive committee—may administer drugs to cause moderate or conscious sedation. The physician may do so only to patients with a pre-procedure ASA score of I or II. Patients with an ASA score of III or greater require an anesthesia consultation.

Individuals administering moderate sedation are qualified and have the appropriate credentials to manage patients should they slip to a deeper level of sedation. Included in the qualifications of individuals providing moderate sedation is a competency-based education, training and experience in

1. evaluating patients prior to performing moderate sedation;

2. performing the moderate sedation to include methods and techniques required to rescue those patients who slip into a deeper-than-desired level of sedation or analgesia. Specifically, practitioners who have appropriate credentials and are permitted to administer moderate sedation are qualified to rescue patients from deep sedation, meaning they are competent in managing a compromised airway to include providing adequate oxygenation and ventilation. (The specific qualifications and privileging criteria for administering moderate sedation are to be determined by the medical staff.)

Sufficient numbers of qualified personnel (in addition to the licensed independent practitioner performing the procedure) are present during a procedure using moderate sedation to

1. appropriately evaluate the patient prior to administering moderate sedation;

2. administer the medications used to produce moderate sedation;

3. perform the procedure;

4. monitor the patient; and

5. recover and discharge the patient either from the post-sedation recovery area or from the organization.

Appropriate equipment for care and resuscitation is available for monitoring vital signs, including heart and respiratory rates and oxygenation using pulse oximetry equipment. A code cart with reversal agents must be available where the procedure will be performed.

Heart rate and oxygenation are continuously monitored by pulse oximetry. Respiratory frequency and adequacy of pulmonary ventilation are continually monitored. Blood pressure is measured at regular intervals. EKG is monitored in patients with significant cardiovascular disease or when dysrhythmias are anticipated or detected.

The patient's response to care provided throughout the sedation-supported procedure is documented in the patient's record. Outcomes of patients undergoing moderate ("conscious") sedation are collected and analyzed in the aggregate in order to identify opportunities to improve care.

Preprocedure responsibilities

The preprocedure responsibilities of the physician are to

1. ensure that a history and physical are included in the record prior to the procedure for all patients receiving moderate ("conscious") sedation. The H&P (see p. 129) should include documentation of the

    a. chief complaint and history of present illness;

    b. physical exam specific to the procedure to be performed;

    c. review of airway, breathing, and circulation;

d. clinical impression or diagnosis;

e. operative and other invasive procedure plan;

f. pertinent lab or test results;

g. current medications and dosages (inclusive of over-the-counter medications and herbal supplements, allergies and all past medication reactions);

h. physical status assessment (e.g., ASA score I-II); and

i. plan for moderate sedation (e.g. IV sedation with monitoring; see p. 130 for suggested drugs and dosages)

2. obtain and document appropriate informed consent for procedure and sedation;

3. communicate the moderate sedation plan to involved care providers; and

4. reassess the patient immediately prior to administration of sedation and document that he or she remains a candidate for the procedure and sedation.

The preprocedure responsibilities of the RN are to

1. verify appropriate informed consent;

2. gather emergency equipment before the procedure and/or administration of medication;

3. establish venous access prior to sedation and maintain it through discharge.

4. Assess the patient's vital signs: baseline blood pressure, heart rate, respiratory rate, heart rhythm, oxygen saturation, level of consciousness, and Aldrete

score, documenting all measurements on the moderate ("conscious") sedation flowsheet.

Intraprocedure Responsibilities

The intraprocedure responsibilities of the RN are to

1. monitor and document the patient's vital signs every five minutes—or more frequently, if necessary. Physiological monitoring is often the only reliable source of assessment information for patients who undergo moderate ("conscious") sedation.

2. assess the patient continuously for changes in condition and/or untoward responses or effects, and immediately report any of the above to the responsible physician.

Postprocedure Responsibilities

The postprocedure responsibilities of the physician are to

1. document a postprocedure/postanesthesia note, including preprocedure and postprocedure diagnoses, procedure findings, complications, blood loss or specimen removed (if any) and plan of care.

The postprocedure responsibilities of the RN are to

1. monitor and document the patient's vital signs every five minutes until the patient's Aldrete score is equal to 9 or reaches his or her preprocedure score;

2. notify the responsible physician immediately if the patient doesn't meet the criteria specified above within one hour of the completion of the procedure

(the nurse shall continue to monitor and document all of the vital signs every 5 to 10 minutes until the patient reaches preprocedure condition);

3. complete the necessary nursing documentation, including a statement regarding the patient's disposition;

4. follow the procedure for postoperative care of patients, when the patient attains his or her preprocedure Aldrete score; and

5. complete appropriate forms, such as nursing progress notes, per order or postprocedure policy.

Performance improvement

The following data are gathered following the administration of moderate ("conscious") sedation in any site within the facility:

- Unplanned intubation
- Unplanned admission or transfer to higher level of care
- Administration of reversal agent
- Chest pain
- Drop in oxygen saturation to less than 92%
- Nausea and vomiting
- Failure to conform to documentation requirements

These data are forwarded to the PI coordinator and the section chief or department chair for anesthesia and action is taken as warranted.

Sample Pre-Moderate Sedation Assessment Record

(To be completed and signed by the physician performing the procedure and/or the physician administering the sedation.)

Age: years Sex: ❏ Male ❏ Female Weight: kg	Patient I.D.
Proposed Procedure: ❏ Side and site verified	Preop diagnosis:

PAST MEDICAL HISTORY (H & P REVIEWED)

No   Yes
❏   ❏...Allergies: _____
❏   ❏...Medications: _____
❏   ❏...Previous sedation/anesthesia problems (including family history): _____
_____
_____
_____

❏   ❏...Previous surgery: _____
❏   ❏...Pertinent medical history: _____
_____

❏   ❏...Alcohol/drugs: _____
❏   ❏...Smoking: _____
NPO Status: _____

PHYSICAL EXAM

NORMAL? Yes No	
❏ ❏...AIRWAY	ASA 1 2 3 4 5 E
❏ ❏...DENTAL	**PERTINENT LAB/DIAGNOSTIC TESTS**
❏ ❏...CARDIAC	
❏ ❏...CHEST/RESP	
❏ ❏...LEVEL OF CONSCIOUSNESS	
Other Findings:	

PLAN FOR SEDATION

Medication: _____
Plan: _____
_____

❏ Post Sedation Plan of Care:
  ❏ PACU   ❏ Monitored Bed   ❏ Holding Area
  ❏ ICU   ❏ Non-monitored Bed   ❏ Home

❏ Patient re-evaluated immediately prior to moderate ("conscious") sedation

Attending Physician	I.D.#	Date	Time

© 2001 The Greeley Company

Sedation/Analgesia: Medication Guidelines

Adult Guidelines

Medication	Dose IV	Comments
Sedatives		
Diazepam	0.1 mg/kg	
Midazolam	0.05 mg/kg	
Pentobarbital	1-6 mg/kg	
Lorazepam	0.02-0.09 mg/kg	
Opioids		
Meperidine	1 mg/kg	
Morphine	0.1 mg/kg	
Fentanyl	0.001-0.003 mg/kg (1-3 mcg/kg)	
Antagonists		
Naloxone (for opioids)	0.01-0.10 mg/kg	Titrate to desired effect (brief duration of action)
Flumazenil	0.01-0.02 mg	Partial antagonism
(for benzodiazepines)	0.4-1.0 mg	Complete antagonism
	0.05 mg/kg	Benzodiazepine withdrawal-induced seizures; residual sedation/hypoventilation

General Cautions:

1. Individualize dose

2. Do not give by rapid or single bolus IV administration

3. Expect individual response to vary with age, physical status, and concomitant medications.

4. Use small increments to achieve the appropriate level of sedation.

5. Wait two or more minutes after each increment to evaluate sedative effect fully.

6. If other central nervous system depressants are used, patient will generally require lower dose than non-premedicated patients.

Reference: Holzman et al, "Sedation guidelines for nonanesthesiologist", J. Clin. Anesthesia, Vol 6 July/August 1994 pg. 273.

SUGGESTED DRUGS AND PEDIATRIC DOSES FOR MODERATE SEDATION			
Medication	**Route**	**Dose**	**Comments**
Midazolam	Oral	0.5-0.7 mg/kg	
	Rectal	0.5-1.0 mg/kg	
	Nasal	0.2-0.4 mg/kg	
	Sublingual	0.2 mg/kg	
	Intravenous	0.05-0.10 mg/kg	
Chloral Hydrate	Orally or Rectally	80 mg/kg Repeat dose 25 mg/kg	Initial dose maximum 2 grams Repeat dose maximum 1 gram
Pentobarbital	IV	Initial dose 1mg/kg	May titrate to a maximum of 6 mg/kg

CAUTION: The moderate ("conscious") sedation policy and dosage guidelines are provided as illustrations only. Individuals and institutions are encouraged to create their own documents based upon their unique practitioner preferences, patient populations, scope of services provided, and other clinical variables.

Sample Consent Form for Anesthesia

I have informed _____,
Patient name

or the person authorized to extend the patient's consent, of the methods of
anesthesia proposed for the planned procedure. I have explained, consistent
with accepted medical judgment, the nature and purpose of the anesthesia
and the reasonable alternative anesthesia methods, risks involved, and the
possibility of complications. In addition, I have explained that the anesthetic
which is proposed to be used is a

[ ] general

[ ] spinal or epidural

[ ] nerve block

[ ] intravenous regional

[ ] monitored anesthesia care,

but that an alternative form of anesthesia may be used if required by
unexpected conditions arising before or during the procedure. I have
answered all questions to the patient's satisfaction and was granted permission
to proceed.

_____

Physician's signature   Date

Sample consent form for patients who have a "Do Not Resuscitate" (DNR) or similar order in their chart or living will

Because the use of anesthetic drugs may produce significant changes in my vital systems, I understand that "Do Not Resuscitate" (DNR) or similar orders will be suspended during my operation or procedure until I have recovered from the effects of anesthesia, unless otherwise indicated below.

_____

Signature of patient or person authorized to consent for patient

_____

Relationship to patient   Date

Sample Authorization and Consent or Refusal Form for Blood/Blood Product Transfusion

I, _____, understand that I may need a transfusion of blood and/or one of its products during my treatment. The risks and benefits of receiving transfusion(s) have been explained to me.

Informed consent regarding benefits/risks/alternatives

Benefits of transfusion include, but are not limited to

 _ elevation of blood level of the product transfused

 _ prevention of hypoxemia (LOW OXYGEN LEVEL) and hypotension (LOW BLOOD PRESSURE)

 _ prevention of bleeding, bruising, hemorrhage into a vital organ, gastrointestinal tract, or brain (PLT transfusion)

Risks of transfusion include, but are not limited to

 _ fever or chills (1 - 3%)

 _ congestive heart failure

 _ major transfusion reaction is unlikely, but remotely possible, and can lead to death (<0.1%)

 _ allergic reaction (1 - 2%)

 _ transmission of hepatitis (0.007 - 0.03%)

 _ transmission of HIV virus (0.001%)

Alternatives to transfusion include, but are not limited to

 _ no transfusion, accepting present condition and risks

 _ donating my own blood (only available before planned surgery)

 _ receiving my own blood back (autologous transfusion)

 _ having someone donate blood on my behalf (directed donation, only available before surgery)

Opportunity for questions was offered.

_ I understand the above information and consent to the transfusion(s) of blood or blood products.

_ I refuse consent for blood or blood products – I understand that my refusal may cause serious harm or death.

_____   _____
Patient's signature (or legal representative)   Date

I have explained the risks, benefits, potential complications, and alternatives of the treatment to the patient and have answered all questions to the patient's satisfaction, and they have granted consent to proceed.

_____   _____
Physician's signature   Date

If this document is not signed by the patient, complete either item A or B below, whichever applies.

A. The patient is a minor, _____ years of age.
B. The patient was unable to sign because

_____

_____

_____

_____

Informed Consent for Operative or Invasive Procedure, Anesthesia/Moderate Sedation, and Blood

Patient: _____ Date of Birth: _____

1. I give my permission to Dr.(s) _____

to perform the following procedure(s)/treatment(s) _____

_____

2. I understand that during this procedure/treatment new findings or conditions may appear and require an additional procedure/treatment for proper care.

3. Dr. _____ has discussed with me the items below, including, but not limited to the following:

A. My condition _____

B. The purpose and expected benefits of the procedure/treatment _____

_____

C. Just as there may be benefits to the procedure, I understand that all medical procedures/treatments involve risk. These general risks or possible complications include but are not limited to bleeding, blood clots, tissue damage, pain, respiratory problems, infections, loss of sensation, loss of motion, and even loss of bodily function or life. I also realize that the following additional risks may occur in connection with the particular procedure/treatment proposed for me: _____

D. The alternatives to this procedure and what could happen if nothing is done.

_____

4. I know that other unexplained risks or complications not discussed may occur and that there is no guarantee about the results of the procedure/treatment.

5. I understand that, during or after the procedure, my doctor may feel it necessary to give me a transfusion of blood or blood components. My doctor has discussed with me the alternatives to, and possible risks of transfusion, including unexpected blood reactions and the possible transmission of certain viruses, including hepatitis and AIDS, however remote.

6. I know that other clinical staff may help my doctor during the procedure/treatment.

7. I understand that the procedure may require that I undergo some form of anesthesia, which may have its own risks. My doctor or a representative from the department of anesthesiology has informed me of the course of anesthesia that is recommended (if any) along with its possible risks and alternatives.

8. Any tissue or specimens taken from my body as a result of the procedure may be examined and disposed of, retained, preserved, or used for medical, scientific, or teaching purposes by the hospital.

9. I understand that my surgical/diagnostic procedure/treatment may be photographed or videotaped and that observers may be present in the operating, treatment, or procedure room for the purpose of advancing medical care and education.

10. I understand that all means of resuscitation will be pursued, should my heart stop beating during the procedure.

11. I impose no specific limitations or prohibitions regarding treatment other than the following: _____

_____

12. I understand what my doctor has explained to me and have had all my questions fully answered.

13. Having talked with my doctor and having the opportunity to read this form, my signature below acknowledges that consent to the performance of the procedure/treatment described above (including blood transfusions and other medical products that my doctor feels are necessary or advisable.)

_____   _____

Patient's Signature (or Legal Representative)   Date

I have explained the risks, benefits, potential complications, and alternatives of the treatment to the patient and have answered all questions to the patient's satisfaction, and they have granted consent to proceed.

_____   _____

Physician's Signature   Date

Anesthesia Guidelines and Standards

This appendix contains standards and guidelines published by the American Society of Anesthesiologists (ASA). Much of this information was published in ASA's *2001 Directory of Members* and has been reprinted with permission.

Continuum of Depth of Sedation
Definition of General Anesthesia
and Levels of Sedation/Analgesia[1]

(Approved by House of Delegates on October 13, 1999)

	Minimal Sedation (Anxiolysis)	Moderate Sedation/ Analgesia "Conscious Sedation")	Deep Sedation/ Analgesia	General Anesthesia
Responsiveness	Normal response to verbal stimulation	Purposeful[2] response to verbal or tactile stimulation	Purposeful[2] response following repeated or painful stimulation	Unarousable even with painful stimulus
Airway	Unaffected	No intervention required	Intervention may be required	Intervention often required
Spontaneous Ventilation	Unaffected	Adequate	May be Inadequate	Frequently inadequate
Cardiovascular Function	Unaffected	Usually maintained	Usually maintained	May be impaired

Minimal sedation (anxiolysis) *is a drug-induced state during which patients respond normally to verbal commands. Although cognitive function and coordination may be impaired, ventilatory and cardiovascular functions are unaffected.*

Moderate sedation/analgesia ("conscious sedation") *is a drug-induced depression of consciousness during which patients respond purposefully[2]*

---

[1] *Monitored Anesthesia Care does not describe the continuum of depth of sedation, rather it describes "a specific anesthesia service in which an anesthesiologist has been requested to participate in the care of a patient undergoing a diagnostic or therapeutic procedure,"*
[2] *Reflex withdrawal from a painful stimulus is NOT considered a purposeful response.*

to verbal commands, either alone or accompanied by light tactile stimulation. No interventions are required to maintain a patent airway, and spontaneous ventilation is adequate. Cardiovascular function is usually maintained.

Deep sedation/analgesia is a drug-induced depression of consciousness during which patients cannot be easily aroused but respond purposefully[2] following repeated or painful stimulation. The ability to independently maintain ventilatory function may be impaired. Patients may require assistance in maintaining a patent airway, and spontaneous ventilation may be inadequate. Cardiovascular function is usually maintained.

General anesthesia is a drug-induced loss of consciousness during which patients are not arousable, even by painful stimulation. The ability to independently maintain ventilatory function is often impaired. Patients often require assistance in maintaining a patent airway, and they may require positive pressure ventilation because of depressed spontaneous ventilation or drug-induced depression of neuromuscular function. Cardiovascular function may be impaired.

Because sedation is a continuum, it is not always possible to predict how an individual patient will respond. Hence, practitioners intending to produce a given level of sedation should be able to rescue patients whose level of sedation becomes deeper than initially intended. Individuals administering moderate sedation/analgesia ("conscious sedation") should be able to rescue patients who enter a state of deep sedation/analgesia, while those administering deep sedation/analgesia should be able to rescue patients who enter a state of general anesthesia.

"Continuum of Depth of Sedation Definition of General Anesthesia and Levels of Sedation/Analgesia" © 2001 is reprinted with permission of the American Society of Anesthesiologists, 520 N. Northwest Highway, Park Ridge, IL 6008-2573.

Guidelines for Minimally Acceptable Continuing Medical Education in Anesthesiology

(Approved by House of Delegates October 4, 1972; last amended October 13, 1989)

I. The program should consist of a minimum of 150 hours of approved postgraduate education every three years.

II. Approved postgraduate educational experience should include the following:

Category I (minimum 60 hours)

The Society believes that 60 hours is the minimum time that should be spent in Category I efforts. We recognize that hours of credit suggested for the subcategories below are quite appropriately subject to some degree of variation from one program to another.

A. An ACGME-accredited transitional year, residency, or fellowship should be credited at 50 hours per year for full-time training. No credit for training prior to the three-year period under consideration should be allowed.

B. Fifty credit hours should be allowed for each full academic year of education leading to an advanced degree other than the MD degree in a medical field or medically related science. Education must occur within the three-year period under consideration.

C. Continuing medical education courses should be credited on an hour-for-hour basis for the number of hours of course attendance. Approved courses should include:

1. Any formally constituted meeting, program, or course taught or sponsored by a medical school accredited by the LCME.

2. Any formally constituted meeting, program, or course sponsored by an institution or hospital accredited by the AMA or State Medical Society.

3. Any formally constituted meeting, program, or course offered nationally or locally by any of the specialty societies recognized by the AMA. This would include programs sponsored by the ASA or its component societies.

D. Thirty credit hours should be allowed for each examination in which a physician participates in the ASA Self-Evaluation Program for a potential 60 credit hours per year.

Category II (maximum 90 hours)

A. Up to 24 credit hours per year should be allowed for hours of self-education by tapes such as those of the American College of Physicians or Audio-Digest.

B. Up to 24 credit hours per year should be allowed for hours of self-education through the study of medical literature related to the specialty.

C. Up to 10 credit hours per year should be allowed for hours spent teaching anesthesiology-related sciences to medical students, graduate physicians, or allied health personnel.

D. Up to 10 credit hours per year should be allowed for hours spent in the initial preparation and publication of scientific papers.

E. Up to 10 credit hours per year should be allowed for presentation of each paper, course, or exhibit at meetings of any national, regional, or local medical group recognized by the AMA.

F. Hour-for-hour credit should be allowed for such educational activities as attendance at:

1. Medical meetings, programs, courses, or scheduled grand rounds not included in previous categories.

2. Postmortems with a pathologist

3. Journal clubs.

The Society and its Section on Education and Research will continue to coordinate and promote the availability nationally, regionally, and locally of suitable continuing medical education activities.

The decision for the initiation of programs for required continuing education shall remain a responsibility of the component societies.

Documentation of Anesthesia Care

(Approved by House of Delegates on October 12, 1988)

Documentation is a factor in the provision of quality care and is the responsibility of an anesthesiologist. While anesthesia care is a continuum, it is usually viewed as consisting of preanesthesia, perianesthesia, and postanesthesia components. Anesthesia care should be documented to reflect these components and to facilitate review.

The record should include documentation of:

I. Preanesthesia Evaluation[1]

A. Patient interview to review:

1. Medical history

2. Anesthesia history

3. Medication history

B. Appropriate physical examination.

C. Review of objective diagnostic data (e.g., laboratory and x-ray).

D. Assignment of ASA physical status (see p. 25).

E. Formulation and discussion of an anesthesia plan with the patient and/or responsible adult.

II. Perianesthesia (time-based record of events)

A. Immediate review prior to initiation of anesthetic procedures:

1. Patient reevaluation

2. Check of equipment, drugs, and gas supply

---

[1] See Basic Standards for Preanesthesia Care (p. 154)

B. Monitoring of the patient[2] (e.g., recording of vital signs).

C. Amounts of all drugs and agents used, and times given.

D. The type and amounts of all intravenous fluids used, including blood and blood products, and times given.

E. The technique(s) used.

F. Unusual events during the anesthesia period.

G. The status of the patient at the conclusion of anesthesia.

III. Postanesthesia

A. Patient evaluation on admission and discharge from the postanesthesia care unit.

B. A time-based record of vital signs and level of consciousness.

C. All drugs administered and their dosages.

D. Type and amounts of intravenous fluids administered, including blood and blood products.

E. Any unusual events, including postanesthesia or postprocedural complications.

F. Postanesthesia visits.

---

[2]See *Standards for Basic Anesthetic Monitoring (Editor's note: p. 147)*

Standards for Basic Anesthetic Monitoring

(Approved by House of Delegates on October 21,1986 and last amended
on October 21, 1998.)

These standards apply to all anesthesia care, although in emergency circumstances,
appropriate life support measures take precedence. These standards may be
exceeded at any time based on the judgment of the responsible anesthesiologist.
They are intended to encourage quality patient care, but observing them cannot
guarantee any specific patient outcome. They are subject to revision from
time to time, as warranted by the evolution of technology and practice. They
apply to all general anesthetics, regional anesthetics, and monitored anesthesia
care. This set of standards addresses only the issue of basic anesthetic
monitoring, which is one component of anesthesia care. In certain rare or
unusual circumstances, some of these methods of monitoring may be clinically
impractical, and appropriate use of the described monitoring methods may
fail to detect untoward clinical developments. Brief interruptions of continual[1]
monitoring may be unavoidable. Under extenuating circumstances, the
responsible anesthesiologist may waive the requirements marked with an
asterisk (*); it is recommended that, when this is done, it should be so stated
(including the reasons) in a note in the patient's medical record. These standards
are not intended for application to the care of the obstetrical patient in labor
or in the conduct of pain management.

Standard I

Qualified anesthesia personnel shall be present in the room throughout conduct
of all general anesthetics, regional anesthetics, and monitored anesthesia care.

---

[1] Note that "continual" is defined as "repeated regularly and frequently in steady rapid succession," whereas "continuous" means "prolonged without any interruption at any time."

Objective

Because of the rapid changes in patient status during anesthesia, qualified anesthesia personnel shall be continuously present to monitor the patient and provide anesthesia care. In the event there is a direct known hazard, e.g., radiation, to the anesthesia personnel which might require intermittent remote observation of the patient, some provision for monitoring the patient must be made. In the event that an emergency requires the temporary absence of the person primarily responsible for the anesthetic, the best judgment of the anesthesiologist will be exercised in comparing the emergency with the anesthetized patient's condition and in the selection of the person left responsible for the anesthetic during the temporary absence.

Standard II

During all anesthetics, the patient's oxygenation, ventilation, circulation, and temperature shall be continually evaluated.

Oxygenation
Objective

To ensure adequate oxygen concentration in the inspired gas and the blood during all anesthetics.

Methods

Inspired gas: During every administration of general anesthesia using an anesthesia machine, the concentration of oxygen in the patient breathing system shall be measured by an oxygen analyzer with a low oxygen concentration limit alarm in use.*

Blood oxygenation: During all anesthetics, a quantitative method of assessing oxygenation, such as pulse oximetry, shall be employed.* Adequate illumination and exposure of the patient are necessary to assess color.

Ventilation

Objective

To ensure adequate ventilation of the patient during all anesthetics.

Methods

Every patient receiving general anesthesia shall have the adequacy of ventilation continually evaluated. Quantitative clinical signs, such as chest excursion, observation of the reservoir breathing bag, and auscultation of breath sound, are useful. Continual monitoring for the presence of expired carbon dioxide shall be performed unless invalidated by the nature of the patient, procedure, or equipment. Quantitative monitoring of the volume of gas expired is strongly encouraged.*

When an endotracheal tube or laryngeal mask is inserted, its correct positioning must be verified by clinical assessment and by identification of carbon dioxide expired gas. Continual endtidal carbon dioxide analysis, in use from the time of endotracheal tube/laryngeal mask placement, until extubation/removal or initiating of transfer to a postoperative care location, shall be performed using a quantitative method such as capnography, capnometry, or mass spectroscopy.*

When ventilation is controlled by a mechanical ventilator, there shall be in continuous use a device that is capable of detecting disconnection of components of the breathing system. The device must give an audible signal when its alarm threshold is exceeded.

During regional anesthesia and monitored anesthesia care, the adequacy of ventilation shall be evaluated, at least, by continual observation of qualitative clinical signs.

Circulation

Objective

To ensure the adequacy of the patient's circulatory function during all anesthetics.

Methods

Every patient receiving anesthesia shall have the electrocardiogram continuously displayed from the beginning of anesthesia until preparing to leave the anesthetizing location.*

Every patient receiving anesthesia shall have arterial blood pressure and heart rate determined and evaluated at least every five minutes.*

Every patient receiving general anesthesia shall have, in addition to the above, circulatory function continually evaluated by at least one of the following: palpation of a pulse, auscultation of heart sounds, monitoring of a tracing of intra-arterial pressure,ultrasound peripheral pulse monitoring, or pulse plethysmography or oximetry.

Body Temperature

Objective

To aid in the maintenance of appropriate body temperature during all anesthetics.

Methods

Every patient receiving anesthesia shall have temperature monitored when clinically significant changes in body temperature are intended, anticipated, or suspected.

Guidelines for Patient Care in Anesthesiology

(Approved by House of Delegates on October 3, 1967 and last amended
on October 23, 1996)

I. Definition of Anesthesiology

Anesthesiology is a discipline within the practice of medicine specializing in:

A. The medical management of patients who are rendered unconscious
and/or insensible to pain and emotional stress during surgical, obstetrical,
and certain other medical procedures (involves preoperative, intraoperative,
and postoperative evaluation and treatment of these patients);

B. The protection of life functions and vital organs (e.g., brain, heart, lungs,
kidneys, liver) under the stress of anesthetic, surgical, and other medical
procedures;

C. The management of problems in pain relief;

D. The management of cardiopulmonary resuscitation;

E. The management of problems in pulmonary care;

F. The management of critically ill patients in special care units.

II. Anesthesiologist's Responsibilities

Anesthesiologists are physicians who, after college, have graduated from an
accredited medical school and have successfully completed an approved residency
in anesthesiology, and, in addition, may have had additional training in critical
care medicine and pain management. Anesthesiologists' responsibilities to
patients should include:

A. Preanesthetic evaluation and treatment;

B. Medical management of patients and their anesthetic procedures;

C. Postanesthetic evaluation and treatment;

D. On-site medical direction of any nonphysician who assists in the technical
aspects of anesthesia care to the patient.

III. Guidelines for Anesthesia Care

A. The same quality of anesthesia care should be available for all patients:

1. 24 hours a day, seven days a week;

2. Emergency as well as elective patients;

3. Obstetrical, medical, and surgical patients.

B. Preanesthetic evaluation and preparation means that an anesthesiologist:

1. Reviews the chart.

2. Interviews the patient to:

a. Discuss medical history, including anesthetic experiences and drug therapy.

b. Perform any examinations that would provide information that might assist in decisions regarding risk and management.

3. Orders necessary tests and medications essential to the conduct of anesthesia.

4. Obtains consultations as necessary.

5. Records impressions on the patient's chart.

C. Perianesthetic care means:

1. Re-evaluation of patient immediately prior to induction.

2. Preparation and check of equipment, drugs, fluids, and gas supplies.

3. Appropriate monitoring of the patient.

4. Selection and administration of anesthetic agents to render the patient insensible to pain during the procedure.

5. Support of life functions under the stress of anesthetic, surgical, and obstetrical manipulations.

6. Recording the events of the procedure.

D. Postanesthetic care means:

1. A member of the anesthesia care team remains with the patient as long as necessary.

2. Availability of adequate nursing personnel and equipment necessary for safe postanesthetic care.

3. Informing personnel caring for patients in the immediate postanesthetic period of any specific problems presented by each patient.

4. Assurance that the patient is discharged in accordance with policies established by the Department of Anesthesiology.

5. The period of postanesthetic surveillance is determined by the status of the patient and the judgment of the anesthesiologist. (Ordinarily, when a patient remains in the hospital postoperatively for 48 hours or longer, one or more notes should appear in addition to the discharge note from the postanesthesia unit.)

IV. Additional Areas of Expertise

A. Resuscitation procedures

B. Pulmonary care

C. Critical (intensive) care

D. Diagnosis and management of pain

E. Trauma and emergency care

V. Quality Assurance

The anesthesiologist should participate in a planned program for evaluation of quality and appropriateness of patient care and resolving identified problems.

Basic Standards for Preanesthesia Care

(Approved by House of Delegates on October 14, 1987)

These standards apply to all patients who receive anesthesia or monitored anesthesia care. Under unusual circumstances, e.g., extreme emergencies, these standards may be modified. When this is the case, the circumstances shall be documented in the patient's record.

Standard I

An anesthesiologist shall be responsible for determining the patient's medical status, developing an anesthesia plan, and acquainting the patient or the responsible adult with the proposed plan.

Development of an appropriate plan of anesthesia care is based upon:

1. Reviewing the medical record.
2. Interviewing and examining the patient to:
    a. Discuss the medical history, previous anesthetic experiences, and drug therapy.
    b. Assess those aspects of the physical condition that might affect decisions regarding perioperative risk and management.
3. Obtaining and/or reviewing tests and consultations necessary to the conduct of anesthesia.
4. Determining the appropriate prescription of preoperative medications as necessary to the conduct of anesthesia.

The responsible anesthesiologist shall verify that the above has been properly performed and documented in the patient's record.

Standards for Postanesthesia Care

(Approved by House of Delegates on October 12, 1988 and last amended on October 19, 1994)

These Standards apply to postanesthesia care in all locations. These Standards may be exceeded based on the judgment of the responsible anesthesiologist. They are intended to encourage quality patient care, but cannot guarantee any specific patient outcome. They are subject to revision from time to time as warranted by the evolution of technology and practice. Under extenuating circumstances, the responsible anesthesiologist may waive the requirements marked with an asterisk (*); it is recommended that, when this is done, it should be so stated (including the reasons) in a note in the patient's medical record.

Standard I

All patients who have received general anesthesia, regional anesthesia, or monitored anesthesia care shall receive appropriate postanesthesia management.

1. A Postanesthesia Care Unit (PACU) or an area that provides equivalent postanesthesia care shall be available to receive patients after anesthesia care. All patients who receive anesthesia care shall be admitted to the PACU or its equivalent except by specific order of the anesthesiologist responsible for the patient's care.
2. The medical aspects of care in the PACU shall be governed by policies and procedures that have been reviewed and approved by the Department of Anesthesiology.
3. The design, equipment, and staffing of the PACU shall meet the requirements of the facility's accrediting and licensing bodies.

Standard II

A patient transported to the PACU shall be accompanied by a member of the anesthesia care team who is knowledgeable about the patient's condition.

The patient shall be continually evaluated and treated during transport with monitoring and support appropriate to the patient's condition.

Standard III

Upon arrival in the PACU, the patient shall be re-evaluated and a verbal report provided to the responsible PACU nurse by the member of the anesthesia care team who accompanies the patient.

1. The patient's status upon arrival in the PACU shall be documented.
2. Information concerning the preoperative condition and the surgical/anesthetic course shall be transmitted to the PACU nurse.
3. The member of the Anesthesia Care Team shall remain in the PACU until the PACU nurse accepts responsibility for the nursing care of the patient.

Standard IV

The patient's condition shall be evaluated continually in the PACU.

1. The patient shall be observed and monitored by methods appropriate to the patient's medical condition. Particular attention should be given to monitoring oxygenation, ventilation, circulation, and temperature. During recovery from all anesthetics, a quantitative method of assessing oxygenation, such as pulse oximetry, shall be employed in the initial phase of recovery.* This is not intended for application during the recovery of the obstetrical patient in whom regional anesthesia was used for labor and vaginal delivery.
2. An accurate written report of the PACU period shall be maintained. Use of an appropriate PACU scoring system is encouraged for each patient on admission, at appropriate intervals prior to discharge, and at the time of discharge.
3. General medical supervision and coordination of patient care in the PACU should be the responsibility of an anesthesiologist.

4. There shall be a policy to assure the availability in the facility of a physician capable of managing complications and providing cardiopulmonary resuscitation for patients in the PACU.

Standard V

A physician is responsible for the discharge of the patient from the postanesthesia care unit.

1. When discharge criteria are used, they must be approved by the Department of Anesthesiology and the medical staff. They may vary depending upon whether the patient is discharged to a hospital room, to the Intensive Care Unit, to a short stay unit, or home.

2. In the absence of the physician responsible for the discharge, the PACU nurse shall determine that the patient meets the discharge criteria. The name of the physician accepting responsibility for discharge shall be noted on the record.

"Standards for Postanesthesia Care" © 2001 is reprinted with permission of the American Society of Anesthesiologists, 520 N. Northwest Highway, Park Ridge, IL 6008-2573.

Guidelines for Delineation of Clinical Privileges
in Anesthesiology

(Approved by House of Delegates on October 15, 1975
and last amended on October 21, 1998)

The following guidelines are designed to assist anesthesiologists and organizations in developing a program for the delineation of clinical privileges in anesthesiology. The guidelines are meant to apply to physicians practicing anesthesiology within an organization that has a formal process for delineating privileges and a program of peer review that evaluates the clinical performance and patient care results of physicians who are granted clinical privileges in anesthesiology.

Anesthesiology is the practice of medicine. Clinical privileges in anesthesiology are granted to physicians who are qualified by training to render patients insensible to pain and to minimize stress during surgical, obstetrical, and certain medical procedures using general anesthesia, regional anesthesia, or sedation/analgesia to a level at which a patient's protective reflexes are likely to be obtunded. Performance of preanesthetic, intra-anesthetic, and postanesthetic evaluation and management are essential components of the practice of anesthesiology.

Privileges in anesthesiology should be awarded on a time-limited basis, not to exceed two years. The granting, reappraisal, and revision of clinical privileges should be in accordance with medical staff bylaws and institutional/facility rules and regulations, as applicable.

To be awarded medical staff privileges in anesthesiology, a physician must fully meet certain required criteria. It is possible to make all the following criteria mandatory or to have a mixture of required and optional criteria. Organizations should determine which criteria to include and whether to include additional criteria based on the institution's individual requirements and preferences. For example, some facilities may decide that certification by the American Board of Anesthesiology is a requirement for clinical privileges in anesthesiology, while others may deem board certification to be desirable but not essential. Similarly, some institutions may decide that subspecialty fellowship training is needed for certain clinical privileges, while others may not. Some organizations may wish to recognize residency training obtained or certification awarded outside the United States. Institutions granting subspecialty clinical privileges may wish to recognize experience as an alternative to formal training in a subspecialty of anesthesiology. Some institutions may wish to modify certain requirements for physicians who have recently completed their residency or fellowship training.

Criteria to be considered for delineation of clinical privileges in anesthesiology education:

- Graduation from a medical school accredited by the Liaison Committee on Medical Education (LCME), from an osteopathic medical school or program accredited by the American Osteopathic Association (AOA), or from a foreign medical school that provides medical training acceptable to and verified by the Educational Commission on Foreign Medical Graduates (ECFMG).
- Completion of an anesthesiology residency training program approved by the Accreditation Council for Graduate Medical Education (ACGME) or by the AOA.
- Permanent certification by the American Board of Anesthesiology (ABA) or current recertification within the time interval required by the ABA.
- Current Physician's Recognition Award of the American Medical Association or completion of 100 hours of continuing medical education

(CME) over two years, of which 40 hours are in Category I of the Accreditation Council for Continuing Medical Education (ACCME).

- Compliance with relevant state or institutional requirements for CME.
- At least 50% of CME hours in the primary specialty of practice.
- Certificate indicating completion of a course in advanced life support within 24 months preceding application for clinical privileges.

The following items are for organizations granting physicians clinical privileges to practice in a subspecialty of anesthesiology:

- Completion of a fellowship approved by the ACGME (critical care medicine, pain medicine, pediatric anesthesia) or by the AOA, or a fourth clinical year (CA-4) or fellowship of at least 12 months' duration not accredited by the ACGME or by the AOA (e.g., obstetric or cardiac anesthesia).
- Current ABA certification in pain management (certificate of added qualifications in pain management) or in critical care medicine (certificate of special qualifications in critical care medicine).

Licensure

- Current, active, unrestricted medical or osteopathic license in a United States state, district, or territory of practice. (Exception: Physicians employed by the federal government may have a current active medical or osteopathic license in any US state, district, or territory.)
- Current, unrestricted DEA registration (schedules II-V) or no history of revocation of DEA registration (schedules II-V) within the past five years.
- No disciplinary action (final judgments) against any medical or osteopathic license or by any federal agency, including Medicare/Medicaid, in the last five years.

Performance Improvement

- Member of an organization that conducts peer review of its members.
- Active participation in an ongoing process that evaluates clinical performance and patient care results of the physician through continuous quality improvement (CQI).

Personal Qualifications

- Agreement in writing to abide by the ASA "Guidelines for the Ethical Practice of Anesthesiology." *(Editor's note: These guidelines can be found in the American Society of Anesthesiologists' 2001 Directory of Members.)*
- No report of any adjudicated violation of ASA "Guidelines for the Ethical Practice of Anesthesiology" or of any adjudicated ethical violation reported by any medical society or medical or osteopathic licensing organization.
- Membership in a county, state, or national medical association or in a state or national specialty society that requires members to subscribe to the AMA *Principles of Medical Ethics* or to the ASA "Guidelines for the Ethical Practice of Anesthesiology."
- Certification in writing that "I am in good health and have no physical or mental limitation, including alcohol or drug use, that could impair my ability to render quality patient care."
- No record of any felony or fraud conviction.

Practice Pattern

- Site of practice is in an office, clinic, or hospital currently accredited by the Joint Commission on Accreditation of Healthcare Organizations (JCAHO) or by the Accreditation Association for Ambulatory Health Care (AAAHC), or that complies with the ASA "Guidelines for Ambulatory Anesthesia and Surgery." *(Editor's note: These guidelines can be found in the American Society of Anesthesiologists' 2001 Directory of Members.)*

- Malpractice claims experience (based on final judgments)—risk-adjusted for frequency and severity with respect to specialty, years in practice, and jurisdiction of practice—that is judged acceptable by the institution's medical staff or peer review group.
- No record of disciplinary action in the National Practitioner Data Bank (NPDB) within the last five years.
- Scope and quality of clinical skills, as evidenced by ongoing peer review, that are deemed appropriate by the organization granting clinical privileges.

"Guidelines for Delineation of Clinical Privileges in Anesthesiology" © 2001 *is reprinted with permission of the American Society of Anesthesiologists, 520 N. Northwest Highway, Park Ridge, IL 6008-2573.*

Sample Educational Material

This appendix contains the slightly adapted text of an educational brochure that Scottsdale North Anesthesiologists, PLC, uses to educate patients and their families about anesthesia care and sedation. This text is the property of Scottsdale North Anesthesiologists, PLC, and was reprinted with permission.

About Your Anesthesia

Editor's note: The following text was developed by an anesthesia group practice for an educational brochure for patients. It is a good example of how anesthesia practitioners can use explanatory materials to educate patients and their families about anesthesia and, thereby, ensure patients are less anxious and better prepared to undergo treatment.

About your anesthesiologist

Each of our anesthesiologists is a medical doctor (MD) who is a trained specialist for administering a wide range of anesthetics and anesthesia services. Some of our anesthesiologists have additional specialized anesthesia training in pediatric anesthesia, neuro-anesthesia and cardiovascular anesthesia.

Your anesthesiologist will meet with you just before surgery

We will review your medical history and ask you about any medication allergies, past operations, and any health history factors or past experiences that may influence your anesthesia. We will discuss the anesthesia you will be receiving. Your anesthetic will be tailored to meet your needs for comfort throughout surgery. You can rest assured that your personal safety and comfort is a priority.

Your anesthesiologist spends all of his/her time during the surgical procedure ensuring your safety. The risks associated with anesthesia have been vastly reduced with new monitoring equipment. Any significant changes in blood pressure, heart rate, or other vital functions are treated immediately. The medications are used very carefully to make sure that your surgical experience is as pleasant as possible. The association of nausea after anesthesia has been significantly decreased with newer medications.

What type of anesthesia should you have?

The type of anesthesia you will require is dependent upon the surgery you are going to have. In most cases, your surgeon requests that we use a certain type of anesthesia that he/she feels will give you the greatest degree of comfort throughout the surgery.

Many operations require a general anesthetic, while others can be performed with a regional block, spinal anesthesia, or intravenous sedation.

Going to the operating room is not a normal experience

Your surgeon, anesthesiologist, and the entire surgical staff recognize the natural anxiety with which most patients approach surgery. We believe a description of the type of anesthesia helps patients to prepare for it.

General anesthesia

When general anesthesia is used, you will sleep throughout the operation with absolutely no pain or discomfort. You will be sound asleep and under the care of your anesthesiologist throughout surgery.

Once you are settled on the operating table, to ensure your maximum safety, you will be connected to several monitors, which your anesthesiologist will loosely watch throughout surgery. A blood pressure cuff will be placed around your arm (or leg) so that your blood pressure can be monitored. EKG pads will be attached so that your heart recording can be continuously monitored. You will be connected to an oximeter, which records the amount of oxygen in your blood. Other monitors are used to gauge your response to medications. After you have breathed in oxygen with a mask for a few minutes, a quick acting sedative will be given through the intravenous tubing.

The anesthetic gas that you will breathe and other medications (given through the intravenous catheter) will keep you asleep and pain free. Once you are asleep, we will adjust the medication for your size and your response to the administered dose. We will continuously monitor your blood pressure, pulse, EKG, and the amount of oxygen in your blood and will remain by you throughout surgery for your comfort and safety. After your surgery, we will accompany you to the recovery room.

IV Sedation with local anesthesia

When intravenous anesthesia is used, you will be sedated and under the care of your anesthesiologist throughout the operation. Once you are settled on the operating table, you will be connected to several monitors.

A quick acting sedative will be given through the intravenous tubing after you have breathed pure oxygen for a few minutes. Once you are sedated, we will adjust the medication for your size, your level of anxiety, and your response to the administered dose. The level of anesthesia will allow you to rest comfortably throughout your surgery. You might feel some discomfort while the local anesthetic is being injected into the surgical site by your surgeon. Once the local anesthetic has been injected, you should not experience further discomfort.

Spinal anesthesia and regional block

If you are having a spinal anesthetic or regional block, your anesthesiologist will discuss the procedure with you preoperatively.

Important things to remember

Any medication that you are taking on a regular basis should be taken on the morning of surgery with a sip of water *unless* you are instructed differently by your surgeon.

Adults should not eat or drink anything for 8 hours before surgery. Unless otherwise directed by your surgeon, please do not eat or drink anything after midnight the night before your surgery. This means absolutely nothing by mouth—not even water, ice chips, coffee or tea, mints, chewing gum, tablets, lollipops, candy, or any other substance. You may have a sip of water when taking any required medications.

If your surgery is scheduled for 2:00 PM or later, you may have clear liquids, juice, or water for breakfast. Please do *not* have milk or drinks containing caffeine, such coffee or tea.

For infants and children under age 12, please follow your surgeon's advice on eating and drinking before surgery.

High blood pressure, if it is under control, will not prevent you from having successful surgery. Please ask your surgeon about taking your normal antihypertensive medication on the morning of your surgery with a sip of clear water only.

Your blood pressure may become elevated during surgery because of medications given or because of stress. Should this occur, medications are available and will be given intravenously to safely reduce your blood pressure.

If you have diabetes that requires insulin, your surgeon (or your anesthesiologist) will give you instructions about taking a reduced dose of insulin on the morning of surgery. Unless your surgeon instructs you on your insulin dose for the day of surgery, you will need to contact your anesthesiologist a few days before surgery. During surgery and the recovery period, we may extract a few drops of blood from your finger to check your blood sugar level and then make any needed adjustments in insulin dosage.

The goals of your anesthesiology team:

- Treat each patient the way we would want to be treated if we were patients
- Patient safety
- Patient comfort
- Patient privacy
- Make your surgical experience as pleasant as possible

Throughout surgery, your anesthesiologist will:

- Monitor your pulse and blood pressure
- Monitor the oxygen in your blood
- Monitor your response to medications
- Adjust medications to your size and your response to medication

After surgery, your anesthesiologist will:

- Accompany you to the recovery room.
- Assure your comfort in the recovery room and administer any medications that will make you more comfortable.

Insurance billing

We will bill your insurance company for our anesthesiology services for those procedures covered by your health insurance policy. You will be responsible for any necessary copayment, deductible, or charges not covered. For those procedures not covered by any health insurance policy, payment is requested one week before the day of surgery.

Anesthesia charges for cosmetic or aesthetic plastic surgery

Aesthetic or cosmetic plastic surgery is not covered by a health insurance plan. To reserve our services, we request that payment for anesthesiology services be made one week before the day of surgery. Mastercard, VISA, money order, or a cashier's check are accepted. Personal checks are not accepted. If the planned surgical procedure extends past our scheduled time, we will bill you the additional usual and customary amount for our services.

Anesthesia charges for infertility surgery

When applicable, we will bill your insurance company for anesthesiology services related to these procedures. You will be responsible for any necessary copayment, deductible, or charges not covered. Many infertility procedures are not covered by health insurance.

For procedures that are not covered by insurance, we request that payment for anesthesiology services be made one week before the day of surgery. Mastercard, VISA, money order, or a cashier's check are accepted. Personal checks are not accepted. If the planned surgical procedure extends past our scheduled time, we will bill you the additional usual and customary amount for our services.

Adapted by permission of Scottsdale North Anesthesiologists, PLC.

Related Products from HCPro

Newsletters

Briefings on JCAHO, Briefings on JCAHO: On-line

Briefings on JCAHO/AAAHC: Ambulatory Care

Briefings on Hospital Safety

Books

The JCAHO Survey Coordinator's Handbook, Second Edition

Information Management: The Compliance Guide to the JCAHO Standards, Third Edition

Patient and Family Education: The Compliance Guide to the JCAHO Standards, Second Edition

Performance Improvement: Winning Strategies for Quality and JCAHO Compliance, Second Edition

Ready, Set, JCAHO! Questions, Games, and Other Strategies to Prepare Your Staff for Survey

Ready, Set, JCAHO! Volume II: More Questions, Games, and Other Strategies to Prepare Your Staff for Survey

The JCAHO Troubleshooter: Best Policies, Practices, and Model Documents for Survey Success

The JCAHO Mock Survey Made Simple, 2001 Edition

The Compliance Guide to the Medical Staff Standards: Winning Strategies for Your JCAHO Survey, Third Edition

How to Develop and Implement a Multidisciplinary Assessment Form

The Privileging Quick Reference Guide, Second Edition

Step-by-Step Guide to Effective Root Cause Analysis

Tough Problems, Proven Solutions: Mastering the JCAHO's Most Problematic Standards

The JCAHO Survey Companion Package

Videos

Rx for Preventing Medication Errors

The New JCAHO Survey: Myths and Realities

Seminars

Effective JCAHO Survey Preparation for the Medical Staff

A Practical Approach to JCAHO Survey Preparation

The Annual Healthcare Survey Coordinators Congress

Audioconference

JCAHO's Agenda for Change Revisited: How to Comply with the Joint Commission's Plan for 2001!

To obtain additional information, to order any of the above products, or to comment on *Sedation, Anesthesia, and the JCAHO Second Edition*, please contact us at:

Opus Communications, P.O. Box 1168, Marblehead, MA 01945
Toll-free telephone: 800/650-6787   Toll-free fax: 800/639-8511
E-mail: customer_service@hcpro.com   Internet: www.hcpro.com
